PRAISE FOR

'An insightful, straightforward yet gentle, and relatable guide to profound self-love and self-discovery.'

VEX KING, author of *Healing is the New High: A guide to overcoming emotional turmoil and finding freedom* and *Good Vibes, Good Life: How self-love is the key to unlocking your greatness*

'*Real Talk* is a wonderful, accessible guide to self-compassion and personal empowerment. Tasha's book is one I will definitely be recommending to clients and friends.'

JOSHUA FLETCHER @anxietyjosh, author of *And How Does That Make You Feel? Everything you (n)ever wanted to know about therapy*

'*Real Talk* by Tasha Bailey is a game-changer. Combining wisdom, compassion and practical insights, she has crafted a transformative guide for anyone on their healing journey.'

ELIZABETH UVIEBINENÉ, author of *The Reset: Ideas to Change How We Work and Live* and co-author of *Slay in your Lane: The Black Girl Bible*

REAL TALK

Lessons from a Therapist
to Help You Heal

TASHA BAILEY

Creator of @realtalk.therapist

RADAR

First published in Great Britain in 2023 by Radar, an imprint of
Octopus Publishing Group Ltd
Carmelite House
50 Victoria Embankment
London EC4Y 0DZ
www.octopusbooks.co.uk

An Hachette UK Company
www.hachette.co.uk

This edition published in 2024

Text copyright © Natasha Bailey 2023

Distributed in the US by
Hachette Book Group
1290 Avenue of the Americas
4th and 5th Floors
New York, NY 10104

Distributed in Canada by
Canadian Manda Group
664 Annette St.
Toronto, Ontario, Canada M6S 2C8

Natasha Bailey has asserted their right under the Copyright,
Designs and Patents Act 1988 to be identified as the author of this work

ISBN 978-1-80419-089-0

A CIP catalogue record for this book is available from the British Library.

Printed and bound in the UK

Typeset in 10/15pt Swift LT Std by Jouve (UK), Milton Keynes

3 5 7 9 10 8 6 4

Publisher: Briony Gowlett
Senior Editor: Pauline Bache
Designer: Rachael Shone
Senior Production Manager: Katherine Hockley

This FSC® label means that materials used
for the product have been responsibly sourced

MIX
Paper | Supporting
responsible forestry
FSC
www.fsc.org
FSC® C104740

There is treasure under your own feet,
if you're willing to dig. It's time to give
yourself the love you've always deserved.

Contents

Introduction   1

1. Feeling and Healing   9
2. Childhood   25
3. Family Drama   43
4. Little You   63
5. Trauma   81
6. What Holds Us Back   107
7. Self-Esteem   129
8. Love and Relationships   151
9. Boundaries   175
10. Body Image   199
11. Sex   217
12. Identity and Justice   237
13. The Ups and Downs of Stress   253
14. Grief   269
15. Trying Therapy   281
16. Final Thoughts: Living Your Best Life   303

Acknowledgements   307
Sources   311
Resources   319
Index   323
About the Author   328

Introduction

'I can't wait for all of this healing crap to be over.'

I was three years into my training as a psychotherapist. All of my emotional buttons were constantly being pushed and to say that I was exhausted was an understatement. The multiple layers of unlearning behaviours were becoming relentless. I had had enough. On this day, I was on the couch with my own therapist (yes, therapists need therapists) and in desperate need of some hope and reassurance.

'At least once I've worked through all my past stuff, I can just sit back and live my best life.'

I leaned back, resting the back of my head on the sofa. I needed to visualize the never-ending glow-up I'd eventually have after hundreds of therapy sessions.

But there was a pause. And when my therapist finally responded, her voice was gentle but the truth of her words shattered me.

'Tasha . . . you do realize that the healing doesn't stop? It's an ongoing journey for all of us. This healing crap is lifelong.'

Her smile was kind and empathetic, like a parent gently telling their child that Santa Claus isn't real.

This was one of many 'Real Talk' moments that I would have in our five years of being in therapy together. The truth was painful but it was exactly what I needed to hear. From then on, I let go of the agonizing expectation I had put on the healing journey to be a perfect trajectory.

Healing isn't always big 'Aha!' moments. It's often small and subtle and revealing, like throwing a pebble into the ocean and realizing something so small can slowly cause ripples over time.

The self-love journey can be long and frustrating, so I'm here to walk along with you

Let me start by saying I'm so glad that you made it here. Since this book found its way to you, it's possible you feel like your past might be holding you back somehow. You might be on a search to try to understand what healing is and what healing you might need to do. You might also be finding your self-love to be challenged by patterns that you've picked up throughout your life, like having wobbly boundaries or choosing the wrong relationships. To unpack all of that, we need to embark on a journey of healing the many parts of our past and present.

Healing isn't linear. It also isn't easy and we can often get stuck in the process. Often healing is about paying attention to where the pain is, and this isn't always comfortable.

But I don't believe therapy and the journey of healing has to be dry or scary or daunting. It can be painful. But we can also tap into joy and gratitude during the process. Healing is bittersweet like that. There can be pain, but there can also be some deliciously joyful, fun, sweet moments too.

Whatever we don't address becomes a mess

One of the main things that we learn in therapy is whatever we don't address becomes a mess. Our past shows up in mysterious ways – be it unhealthy patterns, unmet emotional needs, or the people we continue to attract into our lives – and influences how we relate to others in the world. Until we can unpack our roots and history, we will be haunted by it. It isn't until we have real conversations with ourselves that we uncover what's *really* going on.

Real Talk is my way of communicating and bringing the tools learned in therapy into your hands. This book is a guide to support you to have genuine, authentic conversations with yourself, in order to start the journey of healing your past experiences and cope with the pressures of modern life. *Real Talk* is about having what psychologist Bettelheim calls 'an informed heart'. On this journey, I will be sharing therapeutic life lessons that come up in the therapy room time and time again, so that you can start to heal for your future and love yourself the way you deserve.

Old ways won't open new doors

As a child, I didn't see or have a language for feelings, trauma and mental health. Being of Black British Jamaican heritage, these topics were taboo, despite the various issues in my household. Such issues were hardly spoken about, so I didn't have the words for my story. And so I grew up shutting down a lot of feelings and not knowing how to articulate them. I became a quiet child with big emotions, who couldn't articulate what she was feeling or needing. Though I looked like a good girl doing well on the outside, holding in these big feelings made me feel socially anxious most of the time.

My big feelings followed me into my adult years through my inner child. Little Me wanted to implode. On the surface, people knew me as cool, calm and collected, but beneath that I was bubbling with anxiety and a deep distrust in my own feelings. I became a people-pleaser in my relationships, fulfilling other people's needs because I didn't know how to fulfil my own.

Like most mental-health professionals and advocates, it was my own story that led me to becoming a psychotherapist. Not only did I want to help people resolve their own crap, but I also wanted to learn how to resolve my own. Old ways won't open new doors and so I had to unlearn many of the ways I had learned to survive, so that I could start to live a life that was closer to my best, most self-loving self.

As a trained integrative psychotherapist, I meet a lot of people who were once children with big feelings. But now they are grown-ups with big feelings and adult-sized emotional wounds. These wounds show up as perfectionism, self-sabotage, people-pleasing and general lack of fulfilment in life, love and relationships. Each of these wounds come from something we've survived in the past that never had the chance to heal.

In my professional life I felt frustrated that so many people might never be able to access the deep and fruitful work of being in therapy. And so I began to share my knowledge and mental-health tools through the wonders of the internet and social media — creating a community around @realtalk.therapist for those who want to work on themselves but can't access our overstretched or sometimes expensive services. This book is my way of making the benefits of therapy as accessible as possible by giving you the tools and insight to help you heal and live your best life.

I can never be the expert of your life
First things first, I can never be the expert of your life.

No one can take that place except you. I'm also definitely not perfect or superhuman or fully healed. However, my expertise as a psychotherapist specializing in childhood issues, and my intention to share some of my own pains and mistakes within these pages, will allow me to help you look at your history through the needs of your younger self.

Real Talk is about giving yourself the change to heal from things you usually don't like to think about. This book is not always going to help you feel better. But it will make you feel *more*. When we feel more, we give ourselves permission to feel and release the big feelings that we've been carrying all along.

I have learned how to take my clients to the past to find important lessons of wisdom and I will help you find your answers too. But finding answers can also bring sadness, grief, rage, disappointment, confusion and a hundred other emotions.

By embarking on this journey you will feel deeper, truer and more authentically yourself as you unravel the past in search of wisdom. This is what self-awareness does.

As someone who sits on the complex intersection of being Black, British and female, I don't see mental health and wellness through one spectrum. Instead, I will challenge you to question the role that some of your own identity and intersectionality plays in your mental-health and healing journey.

By tackling the wounds that may have been weighing you down, you will also move further along your self-love and healing journey, acquiring the tools that your parents or teachers didn't have in their toolbox to teach you. Here is a new place for you to be seen and heard.

The journey ahead

I'm so glad to be on this journey with you.

You're the driver of our jeep. You have control of where we go, how far and at what pace. I'll be in the passenger seat, holding the map and giving you directions for where we could go if you're ready. And we have space in our jeep to pick up nourishment and equipment to help you along the way. If you need to pause for a pit stop, do it. If you need to go back a few miles, go for it. If you need to drive past something too difficult for right now, you have full permission. We need to do this at your pace.

It's best to start at the beginning of the book and work your way through. Each chapter is unique in its own right, but they also lean into one another. Within each chapter there are patterns to unlearn and relearn, based on theories I'll share about our emotional and psychological needs.

Healing work doesn't work without doing *the work*. So I have filled this book with moments to pause for self-reflection. **Real Talk Moments** will help you pause and reflect on what we're thinking about. These are full of some big questions, for you to check in with what you're feeling and reflect on your own past experiences. And **Real Talk Exercises** will guide you into a moment of deeper healing, using creative expression, visualization or things for you to feel confident in taking action on in your life. Creativity tells our ego to hush, so that we can focus on saying the real thing, rather than the right thing. It can be helpful to have a journal or a notes app, to help you explore these.

As much as this book is about self-development and healing, you might find it useful to share things that you learn in conversations with the people around you. Not everyone will be able to respect or understand it because it might trigger their own insecurities around their healing or pain. If you're in therapy currently, I highly recommend sharing things that touch something for you with your therapist, so that you can go deeper with that healing.

My clients are my best teachers, and they inspire me to be the best therapist that I can be every day. Throughout the journey, I will share stories inspired by my clients, without using real names or real details, to protect the people I'm so lucky to work with.

For me, Real Talk means real stories, so I've invited some mental-health experts and advocates who have been kind enough to share their own wisdom and stories. I hope they bring you reassurance and compassion.

I will also be sharing some of my own personal anecdotes and things I've learned along my journey as a therapist but also as a human in healing. By being real with you, I hope that I can encourage you to be real with yourself too.

Before we get started, let's check in . . .

Exercise: Hopes and Fears

Take a moment to pause and reflect on the following questions. You could journal, draw or create a vision board of your answers . . .

What are your hopes for this book and the journey ahead?

What do you want to learn about yourself?

What are your fears?

What might you need to let go of?

1

Feeling and Healing

There is no healing without feeling.

B efore we start unpacking our stuff, there's a question you need to learn to be comfortable answering: *how do you feel?*

Learning to say what we feel is one of the first things that we do in therapy. But its so much harder than it sounds.

So many of us live on auto-pilot. We eat, sleep, repeat through our lives without really pausing to feel the feelings we've been carrying along with us. Our lives don't leave much space for our emotions. And thanks to technology and capitalism, there are too many other things that we find easier to give our time to.

But even without that, a lot of us don't quite know *what* we're feeling. Because we haven't been taught how to acknowledge and be with our emotions. It's just not common knowledge. I've met so many clients who have stumbled when I've asked the question, *how do you feel?* We're more able to say what we think will *make people feel comfortable* instead of saying what we really feel.

But doing this only sabotages our healing and self-love, because suppressing our emotions stops us from moving forward. The more we gate-keep our feelings, the more we also gate-keep our healing. There is no healing without feeling. Just like a

wound, what we feel tells us where the pain is. We can only heal
an emotional wound by allowing ourselves to bear and soothe the
pain of it until it passes. We have to feel it to heal it.

On this journey, there will be lots of moments for us to check
in with how you're feeling, as well as what you felt in the past. So
let's start by getting to know our feelings . . .

What actually *are* feelings?

In order to get along with our feelings, we need to understand what
they are and why we have them.

Science tells us that feelings are temporary reactions from
our body. They act like minions who work for our brain, picking
up information from our environment to tell us about our
subjective experience and how to respond to it. They carry
this information from the body to the brain and back again
in a continuous loop, all around the body. This helps us make
decisions we need to make, like who we want to spend our time
with or what ice-cream flavour to choose. Our feelings are like
the anchor to make sense of our experiences. Without them, we
would be lost.

Our feelings tell us what we should approach and what we
should avoid. It's like the difference between coming across a cute
baby and coming across a wild lion. We lean into things that make
us feel safe, valued and curious. But we lean out when we feel
disgust, fear or hate. These signals are there for our emotional
survival.

So what do our feelings have to do with our healing? Let
me start by saying, we all have a bit of a façade which leads to
us hiding our feelings. Something that psychoanalyst Donald
Winnicott called a False Self. Our False Self is our shield, which
protects and defends us against pain, shame and rejection. It
does this by falling in line with learned social norms, fitting in
and control. For example, smiling when we're actually feeling

emotionally rough. We take control by only showing people what we want them to see, like a mask.

That means we also have a True Self – the most authentic, spontaneous, messy and vulnerable parts of us. We are born as our truest selves, and in our early years we allow ourselves to be and feel just as we are. As we grow older, we start to learn from our environment and adapt to the expectations of others. It's normal to have a dance between our False Self and True Self, as they take it in turns to show themselves. We keep our true selves to ourselves and our trusted circle, and show our false selves to the world.

But in order to be our true selves, we need to be emotionally available to ourselves. The more honest we are with our feelings, the more emotionally available we are to ourselves and our healing. The more we hold back with our feelings, the more emotionally unavailable we are to ourselves and our healing.

When we are emotionally unavailable to ourselves, we often invalidate our emotions by thinking things like:

- My feelings make me weak/too much
- It's not good to be so negative
- Think happy thoughts
- Its silly to feel this way
- It could be worse/Get over it
- Whatever doesn't kill you makes you stronger
- Feelings don't matter
- I'm being dramatic.

As my clinical supervisor once told me, if we don't grow up with an openness about feelings, we learn to be scared of them. The truth is, invalidating our feelings doesn't make them go away. It just means we store them up until they spill over and overflow into all areas of our life. And the more we deny what we feel, the more these feelings have a hold on us. Not only that, but when we block the feelings that don't feel good, we also end up blocking the ones that do feel good too.

> **Real Talk Moment:**
> - *How do you respond to your own feelings?*
> - *Think of someone in your life who openly expresses their feelings. How do you feel about that?*
> - *Think of someone in your life who doesn't openly express their feelings. How do you feel about that?*

Checking in

Real talk, are you fine or are you neglecting yourself emotionally?

In my own therapy, it took me ages to learn to stop saying 'I'm fine' each time my therapist asked me what I was feeling. I didn't realize that 'fine' is actually not a feeling. Unconsciously, my false self wanted to gloss over the real messiness I was feeling inside.

Learning how to talk about our emotions is like learning a whole new language. There is a societal expectation for us to be fine and feel fine all of the time. And often a fear that if we were to be truthful about our feelings, we might kill the vibe or make the moment awkward. Our mother tongue might be full of words like *fine, good, OK, all right, blessed* to describe our emotions. But again, none of these are feelings. They're just words that help us avoid speaking our truth, like putting on an emotional plaster or Band-Aid. It is a layer of protection which helps us temporarily and covers up the messiness and complexity of what could be really going on beneath the surface. And hiding ourselves is the opposite of self-love.

So let me take a moment to ask you, how are you feeling? And I mean, how are you *really* feeling right now at this moment? It's OK if you can't figure out what word to describe that feeling as we'll come to that. But for now, describe what's happening in your body at this very moment. You might want to briefly close your eyes to check in with yourself. What is your mind telling you about what you're feeling? Maybe it's busy with overwhelm and confusion. Or maybe it's peacefully quiet. What does your heartbeat have to say about what you're feeling? Is it racing with anxiety or beating with excitement? And check in on the rest of your body. What sensations are happening, where are they happening and what are they telling you about what you're feeling? What are those emotional minions of yours trying to communicate to you?

Have you ever felt swept up by your feelings? Sometimes our emotions can feel subtle, but other times they feel big and overpowering. It can feel like we'll never be able to shake the feeling off. And we shouldn't have to. But there is one simple but important thing that we need to do: name them.

'Name It to Tame It' is super-simple thing we can do to help us not be swept away by our feelings. It literally is what it sounds like: we need to name our feelings to be able to tame them. Scientifically proven by psychiatrist Dr Daniel Siegel, when we label our feelings as what they are, it calms our brain and taps into the parts in charge of problem-solving and understanding. It helps us make sense of things before we start spiralling.

This is why therapy introduces people to their feelings. When we link *what* we're feeling with *why* we're feeling it, we're able to be more emotionally available and loving of ourselves. But to do that, we need to know and connect with the wide range of feelings we have access to and have a sense of what they feel like in our bodies so we can recognize them. Only then can we name our feelings to tame them.

When we are little, we usually know about the most basic of feelings: happy, sad, bad, angry, scared, surprised. Our emotional minions deal with these feelings differently, so they show up in our bodies in different ways.

Feeling	It can feel like . . .	It usually means . . .
HAPPY	Lightness, butterflies in the stomach, can't stop smiling	I'm valued and safe
SAD	Lump in the throat, heavy chest, stinging eyes and wanting to cry	I've lost something important to me
BAD	Sinking feeling, feeling small, time slows down, pit in the stomach	I did something bad, saw something bad or I *am* bad
ANGRY	Tense muscles, headaches, tight chest, hot skin	This is unfair. I'm hurt or my boundaries were broken
SCARED	Stomach ache, heart flutters, feeling on edge, sweaty palms	I'm in danger or at threat
SURPRISED	Wide eyes, still body, numb feeling	I wasn't expecting this and need to let it sink in

We've all experienced these feelings at some point in our lives. But we might have been told some wrong information about them, which still stands in the way of us feeling our feels. So here is some real talk about our feelings:

There is no such thing as a bad emotion
Society loves to tell us which feelings are acceptable and which ones are not. For example, we're often more comfortable showing happiness and joy than we are showing sadness. But there are no 'good' or 'bad' feelings. There are just feelings. All feelings have a purpose and we all have permission to feel them. Just because a feeling doesn't feel good, it doesn't mean that we shouldn't feel it.

Your feelings are not your personality
There is no such thing as an angry person or an anxious person. Our emotions are not our personality traits. Most of the time, our feelings are just temporary. They come and they go. Some might stay longer than we want them to, and we might be going through a particularly rough chapter in our lives. Your feelings are not *who* you are.

More than one feeling can exist at the same time
Sometimes we can feel contrasting feelings at the same time. We can feel many things at once, even when they contradict each other. One of my favourite phrases is the Japanese term *mono no aware*. It's that bittersweet mixture of sadness and gratitude we can feel when something amazing is ending. Like being in a loving friendship group at a particular time in your life but knowing that circumstances are about to change. We can feel happy to have them, but also sad and mourning that things will never be the same again. Both feelings can exist at the same time.

Some emotions work together
Sometimes one feeling can hide another. This can happen a lot if we've been hurt or betrayed. Imagine being ghosted or ignored by a close friend. You'd probably feel angry and confused about what happened, and that might be the first thing you show other people. But then deep down, there might be another feeling. Like sadness or feeling bad, believing you must have done something wrong for that to happen. So one feeling shows itself, whilst the other feelings are in hiding.

Exercise: Feelings Wheel

Now that we're grown-up, our feelings are a lot more complicated than six basic emotions. So let me introduce you to the wide range of your emotions. This is a feelings wheel. It shows us how our six basic emotions can get more nuanced and specific to what we're going through. For example, there are different types of happiness, like feeling proud or content or powerful.

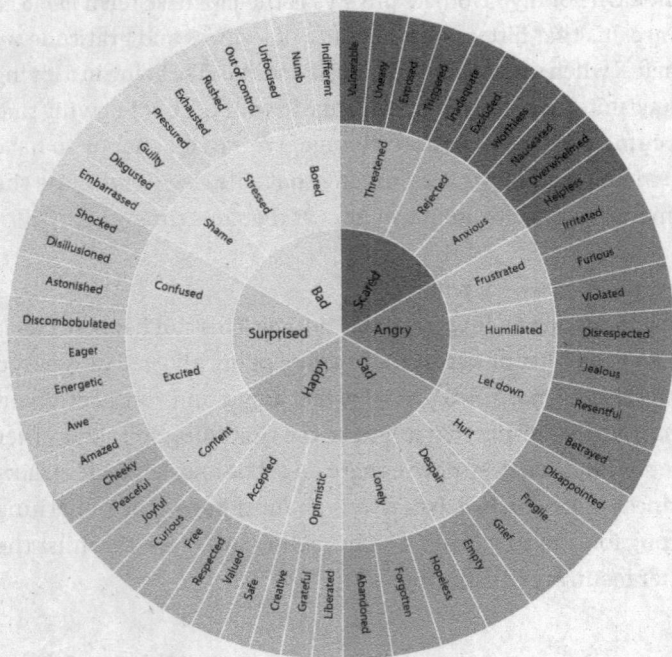

The more that we check in with ourselves, the more comfortable we will be with talking about our feelings. And we're also less likely to feel overwhelmed by them. By using a feelings wheel to check in with yourself regularly, you can open up your emotional vocabulary.

Here are some check-in questions to try:

What word/s best describe how I'm feeling right now?

What does that feel like in my body?

How am I feeling about the week ahead?

What words describe me at my happiest?

What words describe me on the most difficult days?

Feeling unlocks healing

There are sure to be some hard edges of healing. Being on a journey of healing and self-love means we have to come face to face with some tough emotions. It can be a scary and brave thing to confront our own feelings. The difficult thing here is that so many of us haven't been taught how to stay in the presence of our own pain. We recoil when pain and discomfort show up because they scare us.

One of the most incredible things about us being human is our capacity to feel. No other living being comes close to the vast range of emotions that we can feel. And the fact that we feel big, real feelings gives us our capacity to heal from anything we set our hearts to.

A common phrase that we might hear is 'what doesn't kill you makes you stronger'. On the contrary, I believe what doesn't kill you can make you softer, kinder and more resilient.

Many people are terrified of that. To be soft means to be vulnerable and we've been told that this is the same as weakness. And in some families, cultures and groups that softness hasn't been allowed. Having to be tough and resilient in the face of adversity can lead to the image of strength being prioritized over vulnerability.

A researcher in the field of vulnerability and shame, Brené Brown describes vulnerability not as weakness, but as our biggest measure of courage – where we lean into uncertainty, risk and being emotionally exposed. Vulnerability is a choice that we make to be curious and to surrender to the need to be in control. We bravely choose to face scary or difficult things to bring us closer to what heals us.

An analogy that I share about vulnerability with my clients is that it's like letting go of the handrail at a roller disco. Surrendering to the fact that you might fall without it, and people might see you fall flat on your back. But, taking that risk is the only way to grow and get better. When taking those risks of vulnerability, we are able to embrace being scared and courageous at the same time.

When we are vulnerable, difficult and painful feelings will come up. As much as it's uncomfortable, emotional pain tells us where the wound is. Once we know what's coming up for us from beneath the surface, we can start working on it and attending to those needs. It's down to us to be our bravest selves by asking fear to step to the side so we can bear being closer to what hurts us. As much as it is painful to visit where the pain is, going to the emotional places that scare us helps us heal from them.

Being emotionally available to ourselves

Healing is about learning how to be more emotionally available to ourselves. When we give ourselves permission to be vulnerable, soft and messy, we give those feelings the air to breathe. We take a moment to fill our own cup. Because how can we be emotionally available for the other people and things in our life if we're not emotionally available to ourselves first?

Therapy introduces people to their feelings. But there are other things you can do too. Try these practices to open up a more emotionally available relationship with yourself:

- Pay attention to what's happening in your body on a regular basis. Check in with what your emotional minions are communicating to you physically.
- Be intentional by creating pauses in your lifestyle so that you have a chance to catch up with your feelings. Give yourself the gift of your own time.
- Empathize with your emotional needs, not just your practical ones. For instance, a lot of us are more likely to talk about how tired or stressed we are than about our actual feelings. Get into a practice of digging deeper and

finding out what feelings are hiding behind your practical needs.

- Own your feelings by using 'I' statements, instead of projecting or passing your feelings on to other people. For example, 'I feel frustrated' instead of 'You frustrated me' or 'You feel frustrated when'.
- Figure out the root of why you're feeling what you're feeling. Every emotion we feel has a root cause and a back story. Allow yourself to gently trace back to understand what needs to be healed and worked through.
- Notice when you might be avoiding something and allow yourself to be curious about what you're afraid of.
- Give your healing breathing space. It can be tempting to pack our healing journey with different healing methods, because we want to get to our best selves quickly. But healing needs as much pause as our feelings do. Allow space for joy and connection too.
- Allow your feelings to come and go, rather than letting them stick to you.
- Be honest with your feelings, even if it might piss someone off. This might even include ending things and putting boundaries in for people and things that drain you.
- Allow yourself to practise being more vulnerable with people that you trust. But also be respectful of your emotional capacity, and how much of your emotional availability you give to others.

Exercise: The Guest House

A piece of poetry I live by is 'The Guest House' by Rumi. The whole poem is a beautiful metaphor of how we can visualize our feelings as guests visiting our home. Each morning a new guest, aka a new feeling, arrives to visit us.

Seeing our emotions through the metaphor of a character is a method of externalization. In the therapy room, externalizing is when we look at a feeling or an issue as if it is outside of us. We turn it into a person or an object or a metaphor, so that we can actually look at it from an outsider's perspective. We can even turn a feeling or an issue into a character. It might sound a little weird, but when we visualize our feelings as a person, they become something we can have a conversation with. It also helps us empathize with our feelings, instead of seeing them as our enemy. Even welcoming our most difficult feelings can bring us closer to healing the wounds they come from.

Try this exercise to visualize your feelings in this metaphor when you feel them surfacing. You can write, draw or just visualize what comes up. If you feel silly doing this, close your eyes and give yourself permission to be playful.

There's a knock on the door and you go to answer it. Imagine your feeling as the person on the doorstep:
Who is it? What feeling is at your doorstep?
What do they look like?
How does your house guest greet you?
How does it feel to see them on your doorstep? Is there relief, dread or frustration? Note that feeling down, but try to remain polite.

How would you greet them with compassion and kindness? Invite them in.
Give them the floor so they can tell you what they need.
How can you be there for them at this moment? What can you do together that you would both appreciate?
When your house guest feels more settled, feel free to walk them out and say your goodbyes.

The more we make space for all of our feelings, the more space we make for us to heal and grow self-love. When a feeling feels too big, remember you've got this. Even when the feelings feel uncomfortable and the healing feels messy, you are more capable than you know and more resilient than you realize. The more you practise being with uncomfortable feelings, the more you will strengthen your emotional muscles too. Let yourself feel the big and difficult things when they come your way. You'll be surprised at just how much you are able to live through it. And if you're ever in doubt, reach out to someone you trust or a trained professional to walk you through it. But you've got this.

Lots of people come to therapy realizing that the big feelings they have belong to their past. It can be so unsettling to realize we've been carrying emotional baggage for years or maybe even decades. But I think it's great when this happens because it's a sign that we're emotionally ready and available to do the work of healing. We didn't have the emotional tools back then, but we have them now.

And there's one place where a lot of these big feelings come from. Let's take a trip back to our childhood . . .

Real Talk on Feeling and Healing

- We often live on auto-pilot, leaving no space for our feelings to catch up with us.
- Feelings act like minions who work for our brain, picking up information from our environment to tell us how we feel and how to respond in a continuous loop.
- The more honest we are with our feelings, the more we lean into our true selves and our healing. The more we hold back with our feelings, the more emotionally unavailable we are to ourselves and our healing.
- Fine is not a feeling.
- Vulnerability is a choice we make to face scary or difficult things and bring us closer to what heals us.
- We can treat our feelings like house guests who need our time, respect and attention.
- We need to name our feelings to tame our feelings.
- Healing is about learning how to be emotionally available to ourselves.

2

Childhood

Start where your roots are.

People often come to therapy knowing they will eventually be asked to talk about their childhood. And it can be a big question to unpack. Childhood takes up the first 18 years of our life, giving us the most growth and learning of our personalities. So where do we even start?

To make things even more difficult, it's natural for our memories of childhood to be pretty hazy. Our brains are still developing as kids, so we don't have the concrete memory making of adults. But we shouldn't let this stop us. Even when we can't remember solid memories or details in our early chapters, we still might remember moments or flavours of what we were feeling. If we're able to, we can also ask our family members to help fill in some of the gaps. And looking back on photographs can give us some perspective too.

It might be a little painful or sad doing this, because nobody has a perfect childhood. Whether we had a tough childhood or an amazing one, there are always going to be parts that took a toll on us. So starting where your roots are is a great place to begin healing.

The story of our name

Before I was born, my parents couldn't agree on what to call me. My mum really wanted to call me Charlotte. It blows my mind that I could have been called Charlotte. How cool would it have been! What would I have been like? Would I be the same person that I grew up to be? I imagined people would call me Charlie for short, bringing out a more confident and carefree version of me. The name Charlotte also felt undeniably British. What would it have been like to have a name that held so much belonging to the place I was born?

My dad wanted to call me Natasha. A Russian name which means Christmas, and I have no idea why he chose it or why he won the battle against 'Charlotte'. I grew up feeling indifference about my own name. So when I was old enough to go to a new college, I made the decision to revamp my name to Tasha. Somehow reclaiming my name made me feel more myself, affirming who I was becoming.

Our names tell us a story about where we come from. It's where our story begins.

> **Real Talk Moment:**
> - *What's the story behind your name?*
> - *Reflect on who named you, the definition and intention behind your name.*
> - *What nicknames did you love or hate?*
> - *What other things have you been told about your babyhood and the build-up to your arrival?*

Our baby selves

Babies are dependent on adults for their survival. This is the reason why we are so irresistibly cute as babies. From the softness of a baby's hands and bouncy cheeks to their intoxicating scent, this is all a tool created by evolution. Our adorable pull as babies attracts the adults in our lives to become more attuned to our needs. We need our parents to be under our spell as adorable babies because we can't survive without them. No baby can raise themselves.

There can be a lot for our little baby minds to take in. One way that we learn to cope is through 'splitting' our experiences. This is where we draw a line between what feels good and what feels bad. For example hunger for a baby feels painful and bad, whilst being fed feels warm and good. Figuring out what's good and what's bad is how we tolerate overwhelming experiences, and this follows us into the rest of our lives. We quickly decide who we do and don't like at school, the same way we do in our adult jobs. Splitting helps us divide who or what we can and can't trust.

> **Real Talk Moment:**
> - *There are lots of different experiences we would have had in childhood: our family life, nursery, school life, teachers and our friendships, to name a few. As a child, which of these experiences did you label as good?*
> - *And which ones did you label as bad?*

Attachment

How parents showed love and care for us matters. Let's be honest, parenting has come a long way over the decades. It was only in the 1950s that the idea of expressive love and emotional sensitivity began to be seen as important aspects of parenting. This was a pretty radical idea at the time, since the prior belief was that children should be seen and not heard. Before this change, books and experts told parents they should never hug or kiss their children. Growing self-reliant children was the goal. Practical needs were seen as way more important than emotional needs.

It was after World War II that a child psychiatrist and child psychology rock star changed the game. John Bowlby realized that most children were distressed from being separated from their families during the war. Now this might sound super-obvious to us, but it was groundbreaking at the time. It taught us just how much children need and depend on their parents for comfort and emotional safety.

There are five things I want you to know about how attachment works:

- An attachment is basically the emotional bond that we have with someone.
- Our first and most life-changing attachment relationship is usually with our parents, but could also be with a grandparent, relative or guardian.
- We depend on our attachment to survive. In childhood, we need a safe and sensitive adult who can feed, protect and love us.
- We need comfort and safety. To know that a parent has our back, and can attend to our emotional and physical needs, allows us to feel that we are taken care of and not fending for ourselves.
- But we also need space. Space gives us some independence to explore and to learn that we're trusted.

Our attachment is dependent on those early experiences with our parental figure. When we have a safe, comforting and consistent relationship with the adults in our childhood, we grow to have a secure attachment style. It teaches us how to have safe, comforting and consistent relationships with ourselves and other people in our life. If we don't have this experience, we grow to have an insecure attachment style where it feels a little tricky to feel safe and secure in our relationships.

How sensitive our parents are to our needs shapes how we

attach to them. And how we attach to them shapes how we attach to other people too.

A child who feels loved and valued by his parents learns to have love and value for himself. He walks into a room hopeful that he will feel loved and valued there too. Equally, he treats other people with the love and value he's grown to be familiar with. His secure attachment allows him to live and love from a place of security. He can ask for help, be vulnerable and love without fear. Having a secure attachment is having the freedom to love without fear getting in the way.

> In a therapy session with Tally, I had this nagging feeling that she was annoyed with me. It was totally out of character, but that day she was being short with me and avoiding eye contact entirely. 'Tally, what's happening between us today?' I asked. 'Nothing', she said, crossing her arms and looking away. I tried again, 'OK, say what you're feeling.' Tally paused and rolled her eyes before telling me, 'You never replied to my email yesterday. You're never there when I need you.'
>
> I deeply apologized to Tally for not getting to my emails in time, but it also felt like something else was going on here. And when we unpacked it, we realized that she had felt let down by me the same way she had felt let down by her parents. They had never been there when she needed them. Sometimes, therapists can feel like second-chance parents, and in this session Tally was showing me the childhood that she had received. She hadn't felt cared for or remembered, and so her attachment style led her to expect this in our relationship too.

Our attachment can be a bit of a self-fulfilling loop. The more secure we feel, the more secure we are in relationships, which re-affirms how secure we feel. The more insecure we feel, the more it changes how we see and interact with the people we love. And we're more likely to see and do things that confirm that we should feel insecure.

Attachment styles in detail

Developmental psychologist Mary Ainsworth set the tone for our understanding of different attachment styles with her study, 'The Strange Situation'. In this experiment, the mother is in a room with their baby, aged 12 to 18 months. A stranger enters the room and the mother introduces the baby to the stranger, and then leaves the room for the short time. So the baby and the stranger are left alone. Soon, the mother returns and reconnects with the baby. What Mary Ainsworth discovered was that there were patterns of behaviour in how the baby responded to the mother leaving and returning, as well as how they responded to being left with the stranger.

Attachment styles follow us (hello, inner child) into our adulthood. Our friend Bowlby found that a lot of people had the same attachment style twenty years later. In other words, our attachments have the power to stay with us.

However, attachment styles are not a death sentence. Just because we had a difficult start doesn't mean that we can't have better attachments with other people that we meet in life, helping us move closer to being more secure.

Understanding our attachment styles can be a gift. These styles shape the way that we relate to ourselves, others and the world. So let's look at them a little more closely and break them down a little further.

Secure	Avoidant
• Low anxiety, low avoidance • Finds it easy to trust • Trusting, independent and comfortable with intimacy • Communicates without acting out	• Low anxiety, high avoidance • Downplays their relationships and emotionally distant • Avoids conflict and dependency • Acts out by withdrawing
Anxious	**Anxious/Avoidant**
• High anxiety, low avoidance • Difficulty with boundaries • Has a sensitive nervous system • Tends to act out when they feel triggered by clinging or trying to provoke a reaction	• High anxiety, high avoidance • Has a strong fear of rejection • Feels very anxious in relationships and has difficulty trusting • Acts out through self-sabotage

Secure Attachment

A secure attachment is the most ideal attachment style amongst most children and adults. A secure base is a person or relationship which helps us feel safe and secure. A secure base is when a relationship has the capacity to show love, reassurance and intimacy, even when there is distance.

Let's imagine a house party for adults. As someone with a secure attachment, the first thing that we might do when entering the venue is look around and see if there is anyone that we know. We are searching for our secure base. Perhaps a specific friend or friend group. And when we see them, we breathe a sigh of relief because we are suddenly not alone and there is someone at that party that makes us feel safe. We then feel freer to explore the party, to talk to new people and be our more playful selves.

Having a secure base makes us feel safe and confident. In childhood, it's so powerful to know that we are loved. Knowing that we have a parent, friend or partner in a situation who respects, reassures and comforts us is priceless. A person develops a secure attachment when they have grown up with parents who are responsive and sensitive to their physical and emotional needs. They were given space to explore the world and their surroundings, but with appropriate boundaries and support so that they did not feel abandoned. These parents were emotionally engaging and reassuring, whilst also modelling appropriate boundaries and challenges. We internalize the way that we were loved, and this becomes an imprint for how we give and receive love later on. Growing up with these qualities allows us to grow into confident, open and responsive adults, who are able to regulate and manage conflict as well as ask for help. This secure attachment can often give us better tools for when relationship difficulties come up.

Securely attached people and relationships are hardly ever written about or portrayed for entertainment purposes. Because stable and reliable can be pretty boring to look at. Sonny and Cher's ballad 'I Got You, Babe' is a great example of a secure attachment. It describes an attachment which can be stable and consistent despite what they go through or confront in life. In therapy, most of us find ourselves moving closer to the ideal of a secure attachment style as we iron out our insecure patterns of behaviour.

Anxious Attachment

To understand the anxious attachment, we need to listen to some of the lyrics from 'Cater 2 U' by Destiny's Child. The song is full of love and the expression of it through acts of service. However, some of the lyrics step into the area of self-sacrifice and servitude, of needing high levels of intimacy and emotional closeness but to an extent that they may forget that they also need to meet some of their own needs.

In our attachment party, someone with an anxious attachment might cling on to their secure-base friend. They feel anxious at the thought of being left alone, and may follow them to keep close. They may even seek constant reassurance that they look OK.

A person develops an anxious attachment when they have had parents who were unstable or inconsistent with their emotional needs. It's likely their parents were sometimes sensitive, but other times they were inattentive. This gives them an experience of a parent whose behaviour and love is unpredictable. As a child, they were given too much space from their attachment figure, leading them to feel forgotten or rejected. Children who experience this will internalize this rejection and it becomes a deep fear in their relationships. Emotionally hungry, they may have had to fight to be seen and valued by their caregivers. But this can lead to anxious-attachment peeps feeling self-doubt or reacting quickly to feelings and needs. Their self-worth is dependent on their relationships and need for intimacy.

In adult form, anxiously attached peeps can be hypersensitive to the needs and feelings of others. They have developed a hypervigilance to tiny shifts in relationships, and these 'spider senses' allow them to adapt and feel of value to others. They need reassurance and closeness to feel secure in their relationships. Research shows that those with an anxious-attachment style have higher levels of cortisol, the stress hormone, suggesting that their brain reacts more to stress. This would make sense since social hypervigilance – a state of constantly assessing potential threats around you – is characteristic of this attachment style.

Avoidant attachment
There is no better song for describing the tale of the avoidant attached than Beyoncé's song 'Me, Myself and I'. In the lyrics, Beyoncé describes how the only person that she can depend on is herself, and so she banishes her tears and promises to be her own best friend. This is characteristic of an avoidant attachment, where someone has been forced into a position of self-reliance and over-independence. They can have a lone-wolf attitude to life because they've been burned by people dismissing their needs

before. In the Strange Situation, these were the children who appeared unbothered both when their parents left and returned to the room. They instead responded with withdrawing behaviour, such as ignoring their parent.

At our attachment party, our avoidant person acts aloof, standing in a corner as if they don't need friendly conversation. They might even dip out early.

This avoidant attachment stems from not being taught how to attend to their emotions. This is usually because they had to put their parents' feelings and needs first during childhood. They maybe learned that their parents cannot handle their child's feelings and so they protect themselves and their parents by withholding. It's also common for an avoidant to have experienced very controlling or intrusive parents, leading them to feel easily trapped in relation to their parents and others and looking for escape. Furthermore, they may have experienced unhealthy parenting techniques such as the silent treatment, stone-walling or shaming. These experiences lead to dismissing their own feelings and being emotionally distant. Essentially, avoidants learn the narrative that 'When I cry, my parents think I'm too much, and so I don't like it when people get too close.' This internal story tells them they feel trapped by intimacy.

Anxious-Avoidant Attachment
The last attachment style is sometimes called anxious-avoidant or fearful-avoidant. In the experiment, these children showed a combination of insecure behaviours during the Strange Situation. They didn't know whether to draw closer or pull away from their parent. Some people have the tendency to be both.

This attachment style is shaped by trauma and a parent who is consistently unavailable to their child. Having a parent who can be scary at times can be a big influence too. Physical chastisement, or parenting through fear and trauma, can make a child feel incredibly unsafe. A child's first instinct when scared is to run to the person they feel safe with, usually their parent. So it's then conflicting and confusing when the person the child feels safe with is the same person who they need to run from. The adult or adults who should be their caregiver or protector might be the person who causes them the most fear. This can be really confusing for the brain, because our brain will tell us that love and connection are terrifying.

An anxious-avoidant might be scared of intimacy and becoming close with someone, but they crave it at the same time. This can lead to coping through self-sabotage and seeking conflict. They can be hot and cold in their relationships, including pushing boundaries.

We don't need perfect parents

It's best to see attachment as a spectrum that we move up and down depending on where we are in life or who we are relating with.

> *Real Talk Moment:*
> - *What do you think your attachment style might be?*
> - *How do you respond when a new stranger enters the room or enters your life?*
> - *How about when somebody has to leave?*
> - *Do you cling and become anxious?*
> - *Or do you appear aloof and unfazed?*
> - *What are you learning about your own attachment?*

Real talk, we don't need to have perfect parents to be well-adapted adults with 'ideal' or healthy attachment styles. We just need to have 'good enough' ones. Donald Winnicott described good-enough parenting as a parent who responds to us sensitively. This allows us as babies to trust that we can be taken care of, as well as giving us the confidence to explore our independence.

As babies, we are insanely in love with our parents. They are our first true love. We are obsessed with them, and hopefully they're obsessed with us too. But no love is perfect. Our parents might not always have what they need to parent us, which might shape our attachment style. But also, the way *they* were parented and *their* attachment style has a big part to play too.

Parents are hardly ever taught *how* to parent. They're just sent on their way and expected to get on with things. This means that we might not always have good enough parents.

Just like every human, parents go through tough shit too and this can impact their capacity to fulfil a child's needs. For example, a parent who is going through a bereavement or is burned-out at work might find themselves being more authoritative at home than they wanted to be.

Parents can also have different parenting styles for each child. Each child is different and requires a tailored parenting style. Each child in a family has their own unique needs, which can be impacted by their age, gender, physical ability, personality, self-esteem and any neurodiversity needs.

Ghosts in the nursery

Carl Jung says a child's biggest burden is having to carry the unlived life of their parents. In other words, whatever emotional baggage our parents had becomes *our* own emotional baggage. If our parents had a tough childhood, it might leak into ours.

The truth is that the way we were parented, good or bad, will be the roots of our own parenting style if we have children. How our parents were parented impacts how we were parented, and how we will parent. It is as though the unfinished business of our parents in their own childhoods can unconsciously end up on our plate.

For example, in a paper called 'Ghosts in the Nursery', a psychoanalyst called Selma Fraiberg describes a new mother who wasn't able to hear when her baby was crying. They eventually figured out that the mother's own mother had struggled with postpartum depression and suicidal feelings, leading her to be unable and inactive at responding to her babies cries. Having not had a parent to hear and attend to her needs, the new mother unconsciously could not connect with her own baby in the same way. And just like that, history repeats itself. This is of course an extreme example, but with help and support healing was able to take place for both.

This is an example of intergenerational trauma, where the impact of a traumatic experience is passed on generations later. Just like a game of Pass the Parcel, the pain and limitations that one person received in their childhood can be repeated for generations to come. We can see this in generations of families who have been impacted by poverty, domestic abuse, substance abuse, immigration and mental-health difficulties. There are also less noticeable traumas that can be passed on through our parents and grandparents, such as attachment styles, emotional numbness and negative perceptions of children. These ghosts show up within parenting styles, making them more prone to happen again.

For example, some adults from the boomer generation may have been raised to feel that children should be seen and not heard, which as mentioned was the popular societal thinking before attachment theory. They might have grown up without parents who understood, or were able to fulfil, the need for open expressions of love, playful parenting and giving children autonomy. For example, children of the Windrush generation were often separated from their parents during their move to the UK. So there was less time and opportunity for things like play. Or their parents had to take more pride in the practical ways they could provide for their children, with the emotional stuff being disregarded. This in turn would have left those children without feeling emotionally cared for, and hungry for the emotionally nurturing parenting that society now speaks so highly of. This would then impact their relationships with themselves, their partners and potential future children.

In the film *Everything Everywhere All At Once*, we see how this impacts the mother–daughter relationship of a Chinese American family. Their relationship is strained as Evelyn places rigid parental expectations onto her daughter Joy, and struggles to meet her with emotional intimacy instead. Later on in the film, we learn this behaviour is rooted in Evelyn's relationship with her own father who is highly critical, shaming and emotionally unavailable. Our parents teach us to love, the same as their parents taught them to love.

But studies show that when we're in a healing environment, our trauma *doesn't* pass on to the next generation. It ends with us. It is not a death sentence, nor is it impossible to mend. This is amazing news. It means that what we surround ourselves with can be a powerful antidote to some of the effects of intergenerational trauma. When we are aware of our wounds and our risks, we can prepare for them by attending to our healing and the unfinished healing of our ancestors. In the film, Evelyn unlocks alternate realities of herself where she has other skills that were not originally taught to her in her upbringing, which could enrich the way she connected with her daughter and other relationships.

I spoke with trauma psychologist Dr Mariel Buque, who has a special interest in helping people break intergenerational cycles. She told me that:

> a person can be born with a predisposition to high levels of stress and trauma, and will likely suffer a lot emotionally and is more likely to be exposed to unhealthy and harmful experiences growing up. All of that makes for a really

challenging upbringing and creates the foundation for an adult life of emotional ups and downs.

So much of our emotional baggage is captured in the body, in ways that we wouldn't even be conscious of. And it is in the body that we will find a large part of our healing.

Dr Mariel tells us how breathwork, grounding exercises and stepping into nature can help. 'Anything that can help restore the nervous system back to a state of balance is a great place to start. When you've done some of that work, you can then start working on shedding the baggage and unwellness that's captured in your mind.'

Dr Mariel says we cannot heal what we cannot see. We need to understand and unpack what cycles and patterns we're carrying that didn't originally belong to us.

Once you start to notice the patterns, they can be easier to disrupt. And if they are hard to spot, you can always start with acknowledging what feels like it's unhelpful or unhealthy and deciding to do things differently than you were taught. That's a healthy start to breaking the cycle.

A fundamental thing when unshackling yourself from intergenerational parental trauma is learning how to reparent yourself. In order to do this, it's important to connect with your inner child and to learn about what wounds had been left unattended. This can also be great guidance for understanding your parents a little better too.

Exercise: Your Childhood Needs

There are a wide range of needs in our childhood, and it's likely we wouldn't have been able to have all of these met all of the time. Some are practical needs and some are emotional or developmental needs.

Take a notepad and make a note, using this list of needs to think about:
Things I received in my childhood
Things I didn't receive in my childhood

Here's a list of childhood needs to consider:
acceptance
affection
a safe, consistent home
appreciation
belonging
closeness
hugs
community
financial security
access to healthy food and shelter
play
challenge
choice
freedom
independence
space
respect
friendships
safety

stability
to be seen
honesty
trust
warmth
boundaries/rules
consistency
empathy
love
nurture

Looking at the list, what do you notice about what you bring to your relationships, romantic or not?
What do you look for in your relationships? Are there any of these needs that have felt like triggers for you?

One thing I've learned about our childhood is that it is near enough impossible to have all of our needs met as a kid. Parenting can be hard, especially whilst navigating the ups and downs of life. And so parents are inevitably going to make mistakes. But the mistakes aren't what hurts us. It's the drama and conflict that follows that hurt us, and how they are resolved that helps us.

Even though we can't give ourselves a better childhood, we can understand the ways things might have gone wrong, especially in the relationships that we grew up with. And one way to do that is to understand our family life and how family drama showed up.

Real Talk on Childhood

- We learn the most and grow our personalities the most in childhood.
- We learn so much new information in our childhood, so we learn to split everything between good and bad to help us organize our thoughts.
- Attachment is basically the emotional bond that we have with someone, and our most life-changing attachment is our parents.
- There are different attachment styles: secure, anxious, avoidant and anxious-avoidant, which all exist on a spectrum.
- We don't need perfect parents, we need good enough ones.
- Sometimes the way our parents were parented impacts how we were parented.

3

Family Drama

If we don't feel loved by our parents or family, who can we feel loved by?

So many of us go to therapy because of the people in our lives who *won't* go to therapy. Most of all, our family and especially our parents.

The family we grow up with can make us or break us. Our family tribe is supposed to be our ride-or-die pack who protect us and teach us how to survive and thrive. They should be the first tribe where we can fully be ourselves. Where we are loved for who we are.

But our families can also be where we feel a lot of pain, giving us some of the most difficult wounds to heal. How do we untangle ourselves from family mess and heal from the people who should love us from birth?

For some of us, our family pack was the very place where we felt most insecure. This is why some people hate being in groups in general. Think about it, if we can't feel safe and understood in our family pack, how can we feel safe in any other group?

Every family drama starts with the head of the pack. Let's start by unpacking our mummy and daddy issues . . .

Mummy and daddy issues

We don't need perfect parents. We just need *good enough* ones. Good enough parents make mistakes. And when they make those mistakes, they do their best to repair and own up to them. Something that therapists call rupture and repair.

But if we don't have good enough parents or available enough parents to do this for us, we could be left with so-called mummy issues or daddy issues.

Mummy issues and daddy issues are when we have a messy, absent or emotionally unavailable relationship with one of our parents (or maybe even both). Our parents are supposed to be our first true love. They fill us up with the love that we need as children that helps us to become self-loving adults. So when we don't receive the consistent love that we need, it leaves us with a parent-shaped hole to fill. If we don't feel loved by our parents or family, who *can* we feel loved by?

Even when they let us down, we look up to our parents when we're younger. So instead of feeling angry at our parents, we often get angry with ourselves. Parental wounds can make us believe that *we* are the problem. *Am I too needy, too difficult, too unlovable? Or maybe I'm too unsuccessful, too ugly, too far from perfect?* It leaves us with a burning wish to change ourselves so that our parents will finally love us the way we want them to.

Have you ever realized that the person you're dating reminds you of your mum or dad? And not in a good way. Mummy and daddy issues tell us that love is scarce and damaged, and this follows us into our adult relationships. Without knowing it, we find ourselves in friendships and relationships with people who hurt us the same way our parents did. Our brain is attracted to what's familiar, hoping to revisit the same wound but with a happy ending this time. We repeat what we don't repair.

Mummy and daddy issues can leave us with a big, deep hole that we need to fill, and usually with the wrong people, places and things that will add to the pain. If we have mummy or daddy issues, it might show up as:

- Self-sabotage when dating
- Idealizing our friends and partners
- Choosing people in our lives who let us down like our parent/s did
- Using sex to feel loved or keep love
- Trying to be 'good' for other people
- Only dating older people or parental figures
- Believing a partner's love will fix everything
- Constant need for reassurance
- Fear of having kids
- Difficulty with commitment
- Difficulty with elders or authority figures
- Not knowing how to be nurturing to ourselves
- Choosing physically or emotionally unavailable partners
- Feeling not good enough.

Mummy and daddy issues can leave us to feel misunderstood by our parents and we might even struggle to know ourselves. For example, being someone who often gets engrossed in understanding star signs and personality types can sometimes be a sign that you felt misunderstood as a child. Star signs tell us qualities about who we are. We might be looking at these tools in order to feel the connection, reassurance and validation that we didn't feel from our parents.

It's likely that we all have a mummy or daddy issue, even just a little bit. Even if our parents were always good enough, things like divorce, illness or losing a parent can leave us with some big parental wounds to heal. And outside of these, maybe our mum or dad had no idea or no tools to help them be the parents we needed.

Whatever the reason, it's not our fault or our responsibility to be more lovable. And trying to be more lovable in the eyes of someone else takes away from your beautifully authentic self. It may be time to shift the responsibility and let go of any self-blame that you're holding on to. You don't need to change yourself to receive better love from your parents. You are already good enough, just as you are.

> *Real Talk Moment:*
> - *Do you relate to having mummy or daddy issues?*
> - *How does it show up for you?*
> - *What do you think was missing in the relationship you had with your parents?*

How do mummy and daddy issues start?

Sometimes people feel confused about why they would have mummy or daddy issues. They might have had a good childhood with both loving parents by their side. But the question is, how emotionally available were those parents?

An emotionally available parent looks after our emotional needs, not just our material ones. They show empathy and sensitivity to the needs of their children. Just like we said in chapter 2, it ties back to the attachment needs we have. Emotionally available parents make us feel our most secure and confident selves.

Some of us had parents who were physically present but emotionally absent. They may have put a lot of emphasis on meeting our physical needs, like putting a roof over our head and providing for us financially. They take pride in how they can physically provide for their household and this blinds them to being able to give anything emotionally. But this leaves a gap where they weren't able to be there for us emotionally. If they haven't ever done their own healing work, they may not know how to deal with their own emotions, let alone how to parent you through yours. So the moments when we needed them the most, they were not available to us.

Here are some signs that you may have had parents who were emotionally unavailable:

- You didn't feel listened to
- Your parent made you feel that you were too sensitive, emotional or dramatic
- You understood your parent more than they understood you
- Your parent had obvious favourites
- Your parent never apologized for their mistakes
- Sharing your achievements felt anti-climatic
- Communication with your parent was one-sided
- You feel unexpressed anger towards your parent
- Your parent used threats of abandonment, shaming or punishment to parent you
- Your parent seemed uncomfortable with feelings and emotional closeness
- Your parent mostly spoke about their own interests
- Your parent became defensive when you expressed your needs.

It can be lonely to grow up with this kind of childhood. For us to feel confidence and self-love, our parents needed to act like a mirror to us, helping us figure out and validate our thoughts and feelings. Without them by our side, we can find it hard to trust ourselves, believing that we're not good enough. Our parents can become the first and most painful people to break our hearts.

Mummy and daddy issues have us holding on to the burning wish that one day our parents will love us the way we always needed. But we might just be waiting for a parent who will never show up. Sometimes, we try to give our parents (and other people) the love that we were wanting for ourselves. As though we want to teach them how to love us. But we end up overcompensating for the skills they were never able to grasp, leading us to be overly empathetic and talented people-pleasers.

I want you to know that it is not helpful or self-loving to fulfil all of the needs and wants of your parents, just to receive a snippet of their love. If anything, it will hurt your wounds more than it will heal them. When it comes to your parents' capacity to show and give love, you were never the problem.

Love lost in translation

Just because our parent might be emotionally unavailable doesn't mean they don't love us. A lot of the time, it was because they never had an emotionally available parent in their own childhood. How can they know how to attend to your emotional needs if they never had a parent to attend to their own as a child?

But also, sometimes love gets lost in translation. Maybe our parents *are* communicating their love, but not in the way we were hoping for. You might have different love languages. Gary Chapman's five 'love languages' show us that there are five different ways that we like to receive and give love. These are:

Quality Time	Giving uninterrupted, intimate time to doing things together.
	Spending time together as a family: family meals, day trips and holidays, attending parents' evenings and school performances.
Words of Affirmation	Saying meaningful words, positive affirmation and encouragement.
	Saying 'I love you', showing appreciation and empathy.
Physical Touch	Expressing love through non-verbal communication, affection and physical intimacy.

	Safe touch, hugs, kisses and holding hands.
Acts of Service	Helping someone with their material needs to make their life easier.
	Helping with homework, cooking favourite meals, working hard to provide financially.
Gifts	Giving thoughtful gifts and gestures, making the family feel like a priority.
	Celebrating birthdays, family holidays and giving small rewards.

Your love language might be very different from your parents'. For lots of parents who might be emotionally unavailable, things like words of affirmation might not feel like their natural love language. It may feel more familiar and comfortable for them to show their love through acts of service or gifts. Listening out for the ways that they show love can change our perspective about how our parents actually feel about us.

For example, in my family, food brings us together. Our Christmases are extraordinary to say the least, with huge spreads of British and Jamaican dishes, enough to feed every family member twice and still have leftovers for tomorrow. Physical and verbal expressions of affection aren't within our main love language, though that doesn't mean that the love doesn't exist. Instead, we express love to each other through feeding stomachs, banter and fellowship.

When it comes to our own love language, as adults we tend to want whatever we *didn't* receive as children. So if you grew up with a parent who held back on giving you words of affirmation, you will likely look for it in your friendships or dating. It also means that you're more likely to express your love in that way, including to your parents. And the same way you might not be recognizing their signals of love, they might not be recognizing yours too.

Real Talk Moment:
- What ways did your parents show you love?
- What ways did you want to receive love?
- What is one thing you could do to express the love you have for your parent through their love language?
- Could you find a way to tell them about your love language?

Finding parental figures

Whilst we can't go back into the past or change how our parents show their love, we can tap into the warmth and care of other parental figures around us. We can find safe, loving relationships in other places.

> One of my first adult clients was a 70-year-old man called Edward. I was in my mid-twenties at the time, so we found a way to both talk and joke about the age gap and started working on building our relationship in the therapy room. Edward was generous and open to his first experience of therapy, and so many sessions went back to him being a boy, when he didn't have emotionally sensitive parents. One day, Edward smiled at me and said, 'It's a strange thing, but sometimes you feel like the mother I always needed.'

Let me start by saying, this isn't unusual in therapy. It's something that therapists call 'transference', where the therapist reminds us of a relationship we had before or a relationship we needed to have. Sometimes it's helpful, sometimes it's not. But here, with Edward, being the mother he 'always needed' gave him permission to be the little boy in need. We unpacked how he was not allowed to cry as a boy, or during his decades as a man, but how he felt free to cry in therapy with me. His feelings and healing had been unlocked. His tears finally had a place to land.

Not only that, but I worked with Edward in soothing some of his mummy issues by building an internal version of a mother that could be empathetic and emotionally available. So he could be the mother to himself that he always needed.

Therapists can often feel like our second chance of parental love. My actual age didn't matter as much as the emotionally available space that I was providing him. Therapy can be a place where we find these opportunities of second-chance parent figures, but it's not the only one. We can find them in siblings, grandparents, extended family, friendships, teachers and mentors – all of these can be our childhood cheerleaders. Whilst they cannot be our actual parent, they may bestow on us the wisdom, kindness and empathy that we were hoping for, even just in small doses.

As children, we can be so resilient in finding other parental figures around us who can give us what our parents aren't able to. Even if it's just for a few moments in therapy, in English class or at basketball club. It has the possibility of counter-balancing the more difficult experiences we might have faced from our early relationships. In fact these relationships, no matter how short and sweet, help to curate our sense of enoughness.

A Harvard study in 2015 described how children who have experienced trauma can continue to thrive with the help of a caring and supportive adult. It could be a neighbour, grandparent, relative, therapist, parent of a friend or person within the community. I believe this could also come from a religion or scripture. Someone who made us feel safe, stable and valued. These people can place such a powerfully positive imprint on our lives that doesn't go away. We can comfort our mummy and daddy issues by going back to a memory of someone else who made us feel safe and loved. In Maya Angelou's wise words, it's not what people say or do that we remember. What really stays with you is how a person made you feel.

Real Talk Moment:
- *Who was your childhood cheerleader?*
- *Was there more than one?*
- *List the memories that you have connected to an adult who made you feel safe, secure, inspired or valued. What did it feel like to receive their light?*
- *How do you give that light to yourself?*
- *If you can't think of a person, what about an object or place that gives you comfort? Or, for example, a book?*

Sibling rivalry

We can't talk about family drama without the drama that can exist between siblings. Being born into a family means we have no say in who else is going to be in it! Our siblings are literally our ride-or-die relatives. For better or worse, we are set up to spend our lifespan together, especially if we're close in age. Our brothers and sisters can be our best friends, our arch enemies or more likely something in between.

We always fight with the people we feel closest to, so it only makes sense that conflict shows up between us and our siblings. It's natural to feel that we need to measure up to our brother, sister or sibling, or that they need to measure up to us. But sometimes that competitiveness can get in the way of good sibling love.

From the outside, sibling rivalry looks like children fighting over the same toy. Whether it's fighting over a toy, financial possessions or respect, these are just symbols for what we're really fighting for . . . to be loved.

Fighting to be loved by our parents
The minute the second-born arrives, sibling rivalry shows up since both kids now have to share and fight for the attention of their parents. And this doesn't change much in adulthood either. We still want that undivided love and attention. But what makes

sibling conflict really nasty is when we're fighting for the love of an emotionally unavailable parent.

If you've ever watched television shows and films like *Succession*, *Game of Thrones* or even *The Godfather*, you'll know what I mean. The love from one parent may already be so tiny or fleeting that we're left to fight over the crumbs of love they do give out. When the love supply from a parent is low, the competition and resentment between siblings run high. We might be scared that our sibling is more easy to love than we are. We might even have parents who openly compare us, inspiring us to compete against each other. So we go toe to toe with them for the affection of our parents.

But it's important to learn that our sibling's existence doesn't take away the love that is available to us. Our relationship with our parents is separate from the relationship *they* have with our parents. The love for both of you can exist. Your sibling has nothing to do with your parents' capacity to show love.

Fighting to be loved by our siblings

One of the toughest challenges about having a sibling is that we can live in the same family with the same parents in the house and the same school, but can leave with completely different experiences and different opinions. For example, it can be so frustrating to realize that the one person who was our witness during our childhood doesn't agree with our side of the story.

This leaves us with the burning wish for them to validate us, and we so desperately want our brother or sister to respect and relate to us. We're looking for something called twinship, being aligned to someone instead of appreciating our differences. But this need to be aligned just causes friction between us.

Instead of forcing our siblings to agree with us, we need to appreciate that no two people see the same thing the same way, including how they see their own family life. If you want a deeper relationship with your sibling, start with connecting on the good things that you do share together as your safe zone. And then, when that feels OK, explore talking about your differences, without needing to persuade them to change any opinions you personally don't agree with.

Welcome to the family soap opera

Our family home is our dress rehearsal for the wider world, allowing us to explore and be accepted for our personality and quirks. In his book *They F*** You Up*, Oliver James says families are like a soap opera. Each family member has a role they have to perform. Christmas and family gatherings are the perfect example of this. It is almost always the same family member each year who will say something inappropriate. And it is usually the same suspects who turn up later than late. And there's always one person that everyone ends up walking on eggshells for.

It's natural to have roles in our family which help separate us from our siblings. Someone might be the funny one or the sporty one or the responsible one. But if we come from a dysfunctional family, these roles might be a little more toxic. Here are some dysfunctional family roles outlined by author Sharon Wegscheider-Cruse.

	The sibling who is . . .	It's toxic because . . .
Caretaker or Martyr	Looking after everyone else by cleaning up the mess in the family. They also remind everyone to stay in their roles.	They dedicate all of their energy to worrying, supporting and nurturing everyone else in a self-sacrificing way. It also means that everyone depends on them without needing to take responsibility for themselves.

The Hero/ Golden Child	High-achieving and perfect in every way. They make the family look good and represent everything the parent/s love about themselves.	It causes competition with their siblings, and they can be easily replaced if they fail. It's also a lot of pressure being on a pedestal, leading to perfectionism.
Scapegoat/ the Problem Child/Black Sheep	Often named, blamed and shamed as bad, angry or broken. Everyone projects their uncomfortable feelings onto them. But in reality the black sheep is the person who tells the truth in the family.	They internalize the shame and blame, leaving them to not feel good enough. They might even be self-destructive to live up to the title.
Lost Child	Mostly invisible because they make themselves quiet and easy. They keep themselves under the radar to avoid any conflict.	They can be really lonely and self-isolate when they are overwhelmed. They might also believe that they're not needed and not seen by their family.
The Clown or Mascot	The funny or cute one. They help the family avoid conflict by making jokes or changing the subject.	They feel scared of family conflict and as if their humour is all they have to offer. They can be prone to self-deprecating jokes to mask uncomfortable feelings, which is exhausting.

So what happens when we want to hold on to our autonomy and decide to rebel against family roles? Well, the rest of our cast members go into panic mode. Stepping out of the script throws everyone else off course. For example, when the Golden Child throws in the towel of perfection, it can cause an uncomfortable plot twist. Who will be the next Hero for everyone in the family to look up to?

Stepping outside the family lane is uncomfortable. But you

know what? So is staying in it, especially when it's toxic. Just because someone puts you on a pedestal doesn't mean that you have to choose to live there. You are a multifaceted, unique person and you are so much bigger and better than the roles that were given to you.

> **Real Talk Moment:**
> - *What roles fell on your shoulders when you were growing up or now? If you had siblings, what roles did they have? Did your role ever change into something else?*
> - *Friendships are often our second families. Do these roles ever show up in your friendships? Do they ever show up in your work/team relationships?*
> - *If you don't relate, think of your favourite films or television shows with a dysfunctional family instead, like Game of Thrones or Succession. Which of these toxic roles do you recognize?*

Writing your own script

All parents have a toolbox for parenting. But you're an individual, and no tool is one size fits all. So your parents may not have had the tools that they needed just for you or for the context around you as a child. It wasn't your fault and it wasn't theirs. They were using the tools that were passed down to them. It doesn't mean that we're unlovable or need to prove our worth to be loved. But we do need to learn how to give ourselves the love we needed.

We might even be craving that our family members own up to how they hurt us. And though this might feel like a nice way to have closure and how we've seen family drama resolved in talk shows from the 90s, we don't *need* it. Do you need the person that hurt you to tell you that they hurt you? And if you do, what purpose does it serve? Sometimes we only want this because it somehow confirms and validates our own pain. But we don't *need* that to confirm our pain. It was confirmed when we felt and began to process it. Their confirmation of your pain doesn't change it and we don't *need* them to confirm it in order for us to believe it.

That time can't be erased but it can be eased. No matter how old you are, it's normal and human to still want love, affection and recognition from your family tribe. But instead of waiting for our unmet wish to be fulfilled by our family, we need to see and accept them for who they actually are, and accept that they might not ever change. Let go of the fantasy of fixing them and start to decide the realistic capacity for your relationship with them and what that looks like for you going forward.

Sometimes the family drama gets in the way of the family relationship. But you don't need to attend every argument that you're invited to. And you don't need to stay in family relationships that aren't healthy for you either. Put what heals you first.

We're born into families, but we walk into our friendships. We don't get to choose the family that we're born into. But we do get to choose the family we stay with. Friendships are the first place we learn how to be loved outside of our family life. If we didn't feel unconditional love from our families, there's no doubt that we'll search for it with our chosen family.

Through school, work and socializing in different life chapters, we spend a lifetime picking out friendships. And a lot of the time, our family experiences of what we did and didn't have can shape the friends that we choose and the friends that we keep. We find friendships to fill in the places where our family couldn't go.

I call my closest friends my 'sister's from another mister'. We are a sisterhood. Even though they each have a different story from my own, we crave the same thing from each other: the emotional intimacy and words of affirmation. My friends are a place for some of the emotional needs that my family weren't always able to supply the way I needed them to.

A part of writing your own script is finding your chosen family. The family you choose should be the place where you can land as your authentic self.

Traffic lights

In chapter 4, we're going to look at ways of healing your younger self. But it's also important that we decide how to navigate our relationship with our parents in the present.

Letting go of our parents or siblings means seeing them as adults and seeing ourselves as adults too. So when we engage with them now, it needs to be from our adult selves rather than expecting our family members to comfort our mummy and daddy issues or expecting our siblings to be on our side.

Society often tells us that blood is thicker than water, and we can receive judgement for setting boundaries or space from our family as adults. However, when a relationship isn't healthy for us, it's important that we do what is necessary for our healing. The good thing about being an adult is that you get to choose your tribe.

With clients who have had to make this decision, I ask them to think about it as a traffic-light system:

Red light: a closed relationship

We might choose to have a closed relationship with our family if they are causing us harm. Any boundaries that we've set have been disregarded and so we decide to have physical distance or estrangement from them. This can be quite a painful decision for us, especially if they keep trying to contact us.

Estrangement is a little more complicated these days thanks to social media. It means that family members that we decided to distance from may still have access to us through watching our online lives, and vice versa. It means that we get glimpses of their life without us and they continue to have access to ours.

Amber: a private relationship

We might choose to have a private relationship with our family if giving too much of ourselves to them feels triggering. This would involve spending limited time with them. (We might even have a specific duration in mind.) We can also have boundaries around what we speak about with our family members, if we don't trust them with knowing too much about our lives. For example, you might only talk about your job, but not about your romantic relationships or finances.

Green: an open relationship

We might be able to have an open relationship with our family, where we practise openness and vulnerability with them. We feel that we are able to have a good enough relationship with them without losing ourselves in their midst. We can have an adult-to-adult conversation.

> *Real Talk Moment:*
> - *What relationship do you have with your family currently?*
> - *What relationship would you like to have? Is this the same for all of your family members?*
> - *What would need to happen for that to change?*

Exercise: Journal Prompts about Family

Use this exercise to grab a notepad and reflect on your
own family. Here are some prompts to help reflect and set
intentions for your family relationships now and going
forward:
What does family mean to you?
In three words, how would you describe the relationship
with your family currently?
What would you like this to look like in five years' time?
What would need to change within your relationship for
that to happen?
What intention can you set with yourself, to bring yourself
closer to that possibility?
Who do you see as your chosen family?
What words do you wish your parents had said to you while
you were growing up?
What actions do you wish they had taken for you while you
were growing up?

Whilst we can't always take our whole family into the therapy
room with us, we can start the healing work with ourselves and
hope it catches on. Because healing is often contagious. Once we do
the hard work of disrupting the family script, we might just find our
family members going with the new flow of healing and change.

Real Talk on Family Drama

- We all have a mummy or daddy issue, even if it feels like a small one.
- Mummy issues and daddy issues lead us to finding friendships and relationships with people who hurt us the same way our parents did because our brain is hoping to revisit the same wound and find a happy ending.
- Just because our parents don't show us love the way we want them to doesn't mean they don't love us.
- We can find parental figures in other parts of our life, and they can help to heal old wounds.
- Sibling rivalry is natural but toxic if we are fighting to be loved.
- We're born ito our families, but we get to choose the friendships we walk into.
- We might have a family role that we need to let go of.

4

Little You

No matter how old we actually are,
we are only as healed as our younger self.

Our younger self is the part of us that many therapists and healers call our inner child. A part of our personality and authentic self that doesn't grow up.

But this part of us is also the keeper of some of our deepest and richest pain. And when pain is so deep-rooted, it can be hard to put into words or make sense of. Inner-child pain is raw and powerful as hell. It can leave us feeling embarrassed and bashful, because a lot of the time it takes us by surprise and we don't see it coming.

For a lot of us, healing starts with healing the pain of our past. So in this chapter, you will be meeting your inner child and learning how to hold a healthy, loving relationship with them for the rest of your life.

It's time to meet Little You.

Meeting your younger self

For some of you reading this right now, the idea of having an inner child might give you the ick. You may be tempted to breeze through and skip on to the next topic, in fear that I'm about to tell you to embrace your inner child by picking up some play-dough. Now, while play-dough couldn't hurt, my first task is helping you reconnect with your inner child because you probably left them behind a long time ago. Like a little lost child in a supermarket.

The inner child in us is one of the most beautiful parts of who we are. We all have a Little You: a subconscious part of us that represents our childhood needs. Our inner child reminds us to play, dream, explore, be curious and spontaneous. They show up in our humour, when we're with our best friends, when we're feeling creative and even dancing at the club. All you have to do is listen to a nostalgic song from your childhood to be reconnected with the younger version of yourself. Our inner child is the most fun part of ourselves. It doesn't matter how old we are, we carry our inner child with us wherever we go.

Whether we had a good or bad childhood, at some point we all wanted to grow up. In adolescence we naturally start to challenge our parents for independence and we want absolutely nothing to do with being a child or anything that reminds us of the dependency of childhood. (If only we knew how hard adulting really is!) And because of this, we have no qualms about leaving Little Us behind.

Real Talk Moment:
- *When do you feel close to Little You?*
- *When and where does Little You show up in your life the most?*

In the film *13 Going on 30*, Jennifer Garner plays a 13-year-old who makes a birthday wish and wakes up the next day in the body of her 30-year old adult self. She learns that she has everything that she's ever wanted: a great wardrobe, her ideal job and a handsome boyfriend. But just because her body is that of a fully formed adult, it doesn't mean that her thoughts and behaviours are. Her emotional reactions are very much still 13 years old.

This is kind of what happens to our Inner Child. Even though we've grown up, we still have that younger part of us that might take over how we feel and how we act from time to time. It can feel like a button has been pressed and we are catapulted into feeling like a younger version of ourselves. It can feel a little embarrassing to realize that you've been acting 'like a child' in an adult situation. But it happens to the best of us, including me.

An example of this was when I found myself in tears . . . because I had been forgotten in an email chain at work. I hated how childish I was being. Angry and tearful was not what I had imagined for me in my thirties. Yet here I was in raging tears, because of something so small as being forgotten in an email chain.

It was a simple mistake to make, but it had cut me deep. Tears were falling as if they had been waiting for a moment like this. It wasn't about the stupid email, thoughtless as it was. The email was just the 'now story', as my clinical supervisor (my therapist mentor) calls it: stories that happen in the present but have the power to trigger us to the past.

My feelings felt bigger than they needed to be for what happened in the now. Instead, it was about something much deeper driving this raw emotion. Behind it was another storyline of pain, deep disappointment and an unmet childhood need.

These feelings catapulted me into being seven years old again, waiting for my dad to arrive for daddy–daughter plans. I don't know why he couldn't come in the end, but my conclusion as a child was that I had been forgotten. I imagined that he wanted to spend his time with my half-siblings instead and that I was a burden. I remember crying silently, watching the window. I was left alone with my feelings as I wasn't sure if my mum would understand. And so I sat there for hours, soaking in a story of being the forgotten one. Little Me was wounded.

So yes, we all have an inner child. But that day, it was my *wounded* inner child that was in action. The wounded inner child is a 'version' of our inner child. Our wounded inner child is an activist for the ways we were wronged and the ways we were not loved as a child. Remember, whatever we don't address becomes a mess. When our needs are not met or we have deep feelings which were never resolved as kids, they disrupt our development into adults. Those needs remain unmet and those feelings become squashed down, waiting to show themselves again. This is especially the case when we experienced anger or sadness as a child with no one to help us contain or manage it. Instead, we grow into adults with the big feelings of an angry and hurt child. Our inner child has unfinished business. And I don't mean this in the way that a villain would have unfinished business to create chaos and havoc. Even if it feels like our inner child is a menace, they're not. They are just a child: innocent, vulnerable and needing our attention. Their unfinished business is that they need our love and care.

The unfinished business of Little You comes up in our thoughts when triggered. With the email chain, my inner child said, 'Nobody cares about me, I'm forgettable.' It became a storyline for my inner child to hold on to. Other inner child storylines include:

I'm not good enough
I'm a burden
I have to be perfect to be loved
People always leave
I have nothing important to say
I can only trust myself
No one picks me

No one understands me
Everyone is better than me

Something as small as not being added to an email chain, someone forgetting my birthday or being the last one to be invited to an event had the potential to send me spiralling into tears. It taps into my past wounds, time-travelling back to an age where the wound began. When we regress, we then respond from that age, rather than the adult that we are. This might look like uncontrollable tears, a fiery tantrum or rebellious behaviour. Our inner-child pain is showing through. When our inner child is in pain, that pain shows up in our adult lives without our permission or control. We tell ourselves the same stories from our wounded inner child.

Real Talk Moment:
- *Can you think of a time when Little You hijacked your feelings?*
- *How did you feel?*
- *How old did you feel?*
- *What memory did it take you to?*
- *What stories has Little You been carrying?*

Unpacking childhood wounds can be like unpacking a set of Russian nesting dolls. On the outside we see an adult, but as we uncover many layers we might find a screaming, scared child tucked away, waiting to be seen, validated and loved. Exploring my inner-child wound led me to discover several chapters of my life where I had been forgotten, overlooked or neglected. Each had pained me, but I had had no one to comfort me or to help me make sense of it at the time. Little Me was showing me our unfinished business.

So what can you do if Little You is in pain? First, remember that there is nothing wrong with you for feeling the way that you do.

They've been waiting a long time to show you the baggage that they've had to carry. So don't be mad at them for showing up when you least expected them to! Fight the need to rationalize and just be with Little You's story. Take the time to get to know them again and to understand what pain they've been left with. We need to gently find out what wound was triggered for Little You instead of neglecting their needs again. It's finally time to give them the TLC they've been dreaming of.

Inner-child wounds

As Thích Nhât Hanh says, when we cry from deep within our heart, it comes from the wounded child inside us. When our inner child hijacks our perspective and recreates old wounds in adult life in unrelated experiences, we might call that an Inner Child Trigger. It's what Sigmund Freud called Repetition Compulsion, where we unconsciously repeat whatever we haven't yet worked through.

Certain buttons can be pushed that catapult us and our inner child into being triggered instantly. When this happens, our emotions time-travel back to a previous experience of childhood pain. Our adult bodies carry the experience of the little, younger version of ourselves, giving them the mic for how we perceive what's going on in the now story. Some of the signs that we have a wounded inner child include:

- Having big feelings for what seems like small things
- Feeling like there's something wrong with you
- Having a tendancy to people-please.
- Often bottling up your anger or tears
- Fear of being criticized
- Always needing external validation
- Difficulty making or maintaining friendships
- Often going into a spiral of shame
- Fear or hunger to be seen

- Being easily triggered
- Difficulty with authority figures
- Low self-esteem
- Fear or hunger about speaking up
- Perfectionism and over-achieving nature
- Envying or fantasizing about fictional parental figures.

Just like any child, Little You is egocentric (concerned only with their own needs). So when they are hurt, the first thing they do to make sense of it is to blame themselves. So the narrative becomes *I did that* or *It's all my fault*. And so instead of finding the root cause of that hurt, we change ourselves and our nature, in the hope it never happens again. Our inner child is not able to rationalize like we can as adults, so they turn to self-blame instead.

There are four types of inner-child wounds:

Guilt wound

Did you grow up feeling like a burden? If guilt was used as a parenting tool, it's likely that guilt will be a common emotion for you. You struggle to say 'no' or set boundaries and are unable to ask for help. You may attract people in your life who try to make you feel guilty and you may have a tendency to rescue others or have people-pleasing tendencies. This can lead to projecting your guilt and resentment onto others as a way to communicate your needs.

Trust wound

If your caregivers were not able to protect or validate you as a child, you may grow up with a fear of being hurt. This leads to a lack of trust in others, but also a lack of trust in yourself. As a result, you need external validation and rely heavily on your false self to please others in the hope they won't hurt you. You may attract people who are critical or hard to trust.

Abandonment wound

Like me, if you were left behind or forgotten as a child, you may have developed a fear of being left out or abandoned. This looks like an anxiety around relationships and being left alone. You may punish others by threatening to leave, because that may have happened in your own childhood. There may also be self-abandonment, where you abandon your needs in order to fulfil someone else's in hopes that they stay close. You may attract people who are emotionally unavailable.

Neglect wound

Growing up with parents who didn't show their appreciation for you or consistently neglected your emotional or physical needs, you will learn to expect this in all of your other relationships. For example, if your parents never attended your extra-curricular events or parents' evening, you might develop an inner child who believes nobody cares. This feeling of a lack of appreciation may lead to repressing your emotions, but also being quick to anger, as this is the inner child saying 'It's not fair'. You will likely attract people who don't appreciate you time and time again.

	Little You might...	Little You needs to hear...
Guilt Wound	Feel bad or guilty Not like to ask for things or for help Attract people who take advantage of this and make them feel guilt	It was not your fault You did the best that you could I forgive you
Trust Wound	Not trust themselves or others Seek external validation Attract untrustworthy people	What other people think is none of our business Not all people will hurt you I can keep you safe now

Abandonment Wound	Feel left out or forgotten about Find it hard to be alone and is constantly reliant on others Attract emotionally unavailable people	I'm glad that you're here I can show up for you We've got each other
Neglect Wound	Find it hard to say no and to let things go Feel easily agitated and repress emotions Attract people who don't make them feel 'seen'	Your feelings matter Your needs are important It's OK to cry You are worthy just as you

Soothing Little You when they are triggered

Let's be honest, Little You is going get to upset and triggered at times. That's normal but it's also needed. Each time you give Little You the nurture that they need in the present, you heal and soothe their wounds from the past. Our best bet is to be the best parent that we can be to our younger selves. So let's try a reparenting exercise.

Find a safe place to meet Little You. This could be in bed, wrapped in blankets on a sofa, in a playground or in nature. All of these are creature comforts of our inner child. Let yourself cry, shout or hit a soft, inanimate object. When you're ready, ask yourself how old do you feel in that moment. And picture yourself at that age.

Having a compassion script can be useful for any time that your inner child is triggered. Here's an example:

Hey Little Me.
I'm sorry you're hurting. You're safe now. I'm here with you
and I'm not going anywhere. I know it hurts because of what
happened when [name painful experience]. You were only [name

how old you were] and that shouldn't have happened. Grown-ups
let us down sometimes. I know it feels like it's happening again
in this moment, but this time is different. Let me tell you why.
[Explain other possibilities . . .]

Now tell your younger self something that they need to hear.

Little You might need to hear . . .
You are good enough
You are loved
You are lovable
'Perfect' is overrated
I will be a better parent to you than
the parenting we received
I'm so glad you're here
You are a good person
You can come to me when you don't feel good
You can make mistakes

Reparenting your inner child

For many of us, the grieving we have to do for our inner child is
about the parenting we didn't receive but we did deserve. Every
child needs a parent to guide, nurture and protect them. Little You
needs that too. Now, as adults, we can't expect our actual parents,
friends or our romantic partners to be the parent that we needed.
But we're grown-up enough to give ourselves what we needed by
being that adult. Be the love you never received.

Just as we all have an inner child, we also have an inner parent.
This is the part of us who gives us guidance and discipline but
also nurture and protection. Our internalized parent is capable of
helping us with the harder parts of self-care and self-love: creating
boundaries for ourselves, prioritizing our long-term needs over

instant gratification and cutting off relationships that hurt us (which might include our *actual* parents). Reparenting is about giving yourself what you didn't get as a child.

When your Little You is upset or feeling tender, we can show them tenderness and love through our words. By giving them reassurance, affirmation and guidance, we can soothe their wounds and heal what has triggered them from the past. Just like this . . .

> **If Little You says,** *I'm not good enough.*
> **Your inner parent can tell them:** *I don't need you to be perfect to love you. You are always enough.*

> **If Little You says,** *It's all my fault.*
> **Your inner parent can tell them:** *It's not your fault, you did the best that you could. I'm proud of you.*

> **If Little You says,** *Nobody loves me.*
> **Your inner parent can tell them:** *I love you. You're my favourite.*

We can choose to be nurturing, compassionate parents to our own inner child. If Little Us feels neglected, we can comfort them. If they feel abandonment, we can remember them. If they feel guilty, we can unburden them. And if they feel mistrust, we can remind them that we will always have their back. According to transactional analysis psychotherapy, we can have two types of inner parents. We can either have a nurturing inner parent who holds space for our inner child and holds them tight with love and understanding. Or we could have internalized a controlling parent, where we shame our inner child because they don't do what we need them to. This is something we will cover in more detail in chapter 7. But for now, if that controlling inner parent shows up, focus on releasing blame and holding on to compassion. Tell Little You the words that they never got to hear before. This could be *I love you, I'm proud of you, It's not your fault*. Give words of compassion to Little You, but also:

- Read your favourite children's books for comfort
- Create a playlist of favourite songs from your childhood
- Spend time in nature or go camping
- Create a fort and have a movie night
- Give yourself permission to try sensory play (play-dough, bubbles, painting)
- Take Little You out on a date, doing inner-child things
- Returning to a hobby that made you feel good as a child.

Becoming a parent yourself

For a few reasons, our relationship with Little You gets a bit more complicated when actual, real-life children are also in the picture. Having, or even deciding whether we want to have, our own little ones can feel complicated whilst we're also taking care and responsibility for the child inside us. Some worries that I often hear in therapy are:

'*I don't have time for an inner child when I have real children to look after.*' If you already have children of your own, well, congratulations! Now you have one more . . . Little You. It can be challenging to look after your children whilst also looking after your inner child too. You might forget to prioritize Little You. You might even think it's indulgent to give Little You the time that they need. But a healed inner child sets us up to be better parents.

Without healing our inner child, Little You might be pulling our parental strings. Unconsciously, we might get caught up trying to be the parent that *we* needed rather the parent that *our child* needs. It's also common that our actual children might trigger our inner-child wounds . . . which can get messy! And by the way, if we do make mistakes as parents (which we will because we're human), our superpowers of apologizing, accountability and talking it through will save the day. There can be rupture and mistakes, as long as we take the time to lovingly repair them.

Remember that you don't have to make a choice between Little You and your little ones. You can choose both. The activities I listed before to help reparent our inner child work beautifully in the company of the people we love. A day at the farm might be just enjoyable for Little You as it might be for your children (even the older ones).

'Is it weird that I feel jealous of my children? They have everything that I always wanted when I was a kid.'

Ever felt annoyed at your children because they don't realize how good they've got it? It's totally normal to feel triggered because of how loved and cared-for your children are. When we've been let down as children, we often try our best not to let our own offspring down in the same way (though it can happen since we repeat what we don't repair). Envy and jealousy are signs that Little You needs your love and care too.

These feelings can especially come up when we watch our parents be better as grandparents to our own children. Having more hindsight and years under their belt, our parents can mature into being the most incredible grandparents. And this can be hard to watch. This is grief showing up. Not only do we need to grieve that loss, but to be proud of ourselves and the love that we've been able to pour into our children.

'I feel too scared and damaged to have children. What if I'm just like my parents?'
If you're unsure whether you want children, that's OK too. Sometimes people decide this because of the childhood they had themselves. Because they're scared that they're too 'damaged' or not 'parent material'.

However, your history doesn't have to be your destiny. The fact that you have selected this book is proof of that, and shows your willingness to reflect, heal and grow. Reading has already made a change to the blueprint you grew up with. The brain chemistry is already firing up and changing. And though healing your inner child can feel hard, it teaches you not only how to be a warm, supportive adult to Little You but also to future children, if you decide to have them.

Whether we choose to have children or not, healing our inner child is at the heart of healing our selves, making us better equipped to love others in our lives. We need our inner child, just as much as they need us. We are bonded to our inner child for the rest of our lives, and so we should be. Our younger selves give us life, wonder, compassion and creativity. And they always, always bring us unfinished business.

Eventually you'll start to see and respond to your inner child in real time, holding them tight when a deep wound gets triggered. Practice makes this stronger, so keep returning to this chapter and these exercises as time goes on. We will come back to our inner child throughout the book, so keep holding their hand.

Exercise: A Love Letter for Your Inner Child

There will inevitably be times when we leave our Little You behind again. We might be unkind by telling ourselves to 'grow up' or to stop being 'dramatic', or we might even ignore our inner child's needs altogether. But Little You is so deserving of a life of feeling loved, enjoyed and protected. It's not their fault and it's not yours either . . . Mistakes are bound to happen when we're in a place of learning.

When you notice this happening, bring yourself back to them with playfulness. Creativity and play are the mother tongue of our inner child. As children, we loved to draw or write letters, so let's use this as a creative exercise to give your inner child some much-needed love.

Find a safe space where you can't be disturbed. If you find yourself in your head before you begin, jot these distracting thoughts down on a separate piece of paper. Your critical inner parent or shamed inner child might be active and in need of some space to vent. Write down all of the doubts, fears and judgements that are propping up, and when you're done scrunch them up and throw them in the bin. You don't need to carry them with you.

If possible, find some photographs of the younger you. This could be a collection of images of you at various ages, or it might be a particular time period. Do what you feel most ready for at this time. Spend some time observing Little You in those images:

How does Little You seem in the image?

What do you imagine they're feeling?

What was happening in your life at the time? What would it have been like to experience that at the age they were? What did they miss out on? Did you know this at the time or later on?
How does it feel to observe the younger you and to know what you have gone through since then?

Allow yourself to sit with these thoughts and feelings, or journal them.

Next, use a fresh piece of paper to write a love letter to your younger self. You can start by acknowledging their experiences of loss, pain and disappointment, no matter how big and small. You are solely here to validate their experience. If you notice yourself cringing or wanting to dismiss them, be honest by apologizing to Little You and tell them that you're learning to do better by them but it might take some time.

In your own way, communicate your love and care for your inner child and how you hope to express that going forward. Thank Little You for any qualities about them that you admire. Share some of your own words of wisdom with them, now that you've seen what happens next. You can keep this letter sealed in an envelope.

Your inner child had to exist without an ally, and they now have you. How lucky you both are to finally have found each other!

Real Talk on Little You

- We all have a Little You: a subconscious part of us that represents our childhood needs.
- Little You can get triggered by past wounds.
- Our wounded inner child lets us know ways we were wronged and not loved as a child.
- Little You might be carrying wounds of guilt, neglect, trust or abandonment.
- We can heal by practising being the adult that Little You always needed.
- Having your own children can make the relationship with Little You more complicated.
- Playfulness can bring us back to Little You when we need it.

5

Trauma

Something doesn't have to be dramatic to be traumatic.

No story comes without dark and difficult chapters. As human beings, we go through some tough shit, and the word 'trauma' can be difficult to talk about. However, what we go through are the foundations for who we become. So, despite the discomfort and undeserved shame that comes with talking about the darker parts of our story, we have to honour the version of ourselves that had to go through it.

When we've gone through something traumatic, things change. It's like entering your own home and finding the furniture has been tipped over and thrown around. It disrupts our safety and sense of home. And then we have the task of rearranging the furniture to accommodate our needs after what happened. It is hard, but with the right support and compassion it's always possible to create a feeling of home again.

The word 'trauma' has become part of our everyday language. However, not enough of us actually understand what trauma is and how it plays a part in who we become.

So wtf is trauma?

Going back to basics, the word 'trauma' comes from the Greek word meaning 'a wound, a hurt; a defeat'.

Personally, I describe trauma as an emotional wound. Something has happened to hurt us in some way, and we're left to cope with the pain of it ourselves. Sometimes we're able to get help to support us in attending to our wounds. But a lot of the time, we don't have that support, or life moves too quickly to be able to devote time to our own healing. When this happens, sadly it can cause a lot more discomfort and do a lot more damage.

I mean, imagine trying to navigate life with a broken arm and no support to help you heal it. This could make the injury worse and create more difficulties in other parts of your body. Trying to move through life with an unattended physical injury will put a lot of strain on other parts of your body. This is the same with unhealed emotional trauma. Trauma grows when we don't heal it.

Despite what people think, trauma isn't always about one specific event. What makes it a trauma is the aftershock of what happened: *how* it impacted us. Trauma is the scar that is left behind when we are hurt, abandoned or put into a scary situation.

Trauma occurs when a distressing event leaves a lasting emotional response. It disrupts our natural storyline and forces us to find ways to adapt. According to Francine Shapiro, the creator of Eye Movement Desensitization Reprocessing treatment (EMDR: a form of psychotherapy that helps you process and recover from past experiences), we can place these trauma events into two categories: Big T and Small T traumas.

Big Trauma, or Big T, relates to the emotional reaction to a singular event or experience where we survive or witness a physically harmful or life-threatening event. In the same way that a car crash would put our body into shock and potentially cause physical damage, it would also cause emotional shock and pain.

When we think of Big T events, we envisage things like surviving war, accidents, assault or the death of a loved one.

However, something doesn't have to be dramatic to be traumatic. Small T traumas aren't life-threatening, but they are personally distressing. By this, I mean that they may bring up threatening feelings of fear, helplessness, loss, shame, rejection or abandonment. Common examples include break-ups, financial issues, moving schools/house, racial discrimination. In fact, plenty of us experienced a Small T trauma in the form of the pandemic. So many of us were socially isolated whilst inhaling fearful messages from the news, bringing uncertainty, stress, loneliness and unpredictability to our normal lives. For those of us who experienced the loss of a loved one from the pandemic, this would have brought a Big T trauma along with it.

One of my favourite quotes that feels relevant here is 'If you think you're too small to have an impact, try going to bed with a mosquito'. Though they have been labelled as 'small', these types of trauma can be small but mighty, especially when met with frequency. In fact, recent science shows how 'smaller' traumas that happen consistently over a long time period can be just as damaging as a singular, highly traumatic event. Small traumas can grow into big consequences.

Imagine a child was told by a classmate that they are 'annoying'. As a singular event, it sounds innocent and part of primary-school banter. However, if this name-calling is frequently repeated for the same child, it shifts from school banter to a pattern of bullying and humiliation. That child may grow to internalize that message and begin to believe everything they do is annoying. They might start to believe they are an inconvenience, and so resist taking up space or taking social risks. In essence, it diverts them from the normal course of their development. A small but mighty trauma.

Emotional wounds can happen in different ways. Whether we go through Big T or Small T, our trauma stories are valid and unique. It's not necessary or helpful to compare or minimize our trauma wounds against somebody else's. Trauma needs compassion, not comparison.

Childhood trauma

Childhood trauma is something we see a lot of in fairy tales and folk tales. Hansel and Gretel are left in the woods by their parents and meet the wicked witch who wants to eat them. Cinderella is worked to the bone while being bullied by her stepmother and ugly stepsisters. And Goldilocks might have been a child desperate for something to eat and somewhere to sleep. Childhood trauma is more common than we know. In earlier chapters, we looked at how we need a good enough childhood to avoid having a wounded inner child. Children internalize their surroundings and so an emotionally safe home nurtures an emotionally equipped child. However, when there's trauma close by, this begins to shape how children grow.

From a young age, I grew up with a family member with schizophrenia. Though their mental health was usually pretty balanced, it was always the difficult moments that left the strongest impression. Because of those difficult moments, I learned that our household was unpredictable and that feeling safe and grounded wasn't guaranteed. Even though I was never harmed, growing up in a chaotic environment meant that I grew to expect chaos. It's one of the reasons why I became a quiet child, to help keep me hypervigilant to my environment. I became quite skilled in reading the body language of other people – to be ready in case their mood might shift. And in some ways, it probably led me to the path of becoming a psychotherapist.

Trauma is hard enough, but experiencing trauma as a child can be extra-tough on us. The brain is developing a lot in those early years, and so highly stressful events can get in the way of our physical, mental and social health, and of course our attachments.

As an adult, I can see how my hypervigilance held me back from feeling safe with other people when I was growing up.

Childhood traumas like mine are often referred to as ACEs, Adverse Childhood Experiences. When a child or teenager has their trust, security, attachment or boundaries broken, it has the potential to be damaging. An ACE score tells us how much childhood trauma we've had in our story through ten questions measuring the most common types of childhood trauma.

The ten ACEs are:

- Emotional abuse
- Physical abuse
- Sexual abuse
- Emotional neglect
- Physical neglect or poverty
- Parental separation or divorce
- Exposure to domestic violence
- Living with someone with an addiction to drugs or alcohol
- Living with someone with severe mental-health issues
- Losing a parent from death, abandonment or incarceration.

All of these ACEs have a common thread: they can shift the quality of love and care that we receive as kids. Little You learns that adults can't be there for you the way that you need them to be. And because as children we are developmentally egocentric, our first response is usually to blame ourselves when things go wrong at home. For example, it is common for young children going through divorce to believe they need to be better behaved in order to get their parents back together again. But if this is something you experienced, what happened was never your fault or your responsibility. You were just a child in need of love and care.

Childhood trauma is so complex and often comes in layers.

Exercise: The Trauma Backpack

Carrying trauma can be like carrying a heavy backpack. Imagine or draw your own trauma backpack. And reflect on the following:

What does your trauma bag look like? How durable is it?

Do you have an idea of what is inside your backpack?

How long have you been carrying it for?

How has it felt to carry it? How would it feel to rest?

Has anyone else helped you carry the load?

What would you like to let go of?

What is inside your trauma backpack that doesn't belong to you?

What else are you carrying?

What other memories or feelings does it trigger?

The trauma brain

Your brain is a beautiful thing. When things were tough, your brain did what it could to protect and look after you.

To really understand trauma, we need to understand a few things about the brain. Trauma experts Dan Siegel and Tina Payne Bryson describe the trauma brain as a two-storey house. I often expand this metaphor with my clients to help them understand their own trauma brains. Let's take a tour of our house . . .

Downstairs, we have the rooms which cater to our most basic needs: the kitchen, toilet and living room. This is where we feel hunger, exhaustion and comfort. This downstairs part of our brain is called the reptilian brain and is in place from birth, so we can imagine it as the place where we meet our most basic survival needs. Just as a baby needs to be fed, watered, cleaned and comforted to sleep, so do we as adults. So when we're grouchy or 'hangry', this is the part of the brain that is feeling it.

Also downstairs, we have an alarm system which senses whether we are safe or not. In the brain, this is called the amygdala. It is fully installed from birth and it doesn't change from that point. Its purpose is to deal with fear. It acts as a security alarm system to protect us from danger and threat. It does this by working out information sent from our senses and alerts us when there's an intrusion on our safety. An alarm goes out to our body so we can react to protect ourselves. A common action from our alarm system is to release adrenaline and cortisol (a stress hormone) into our body. These hormones kickstart our body into action so that we can attack/work (fight) or run to safety (flight).

For example, if we were to smell smoke, our amygdala would believe there is a fire near by and communicate to our body to find safety. Once the stressful event is over, the cortisol and adrenaline reduce and our body chills out again. However, if we have experienced a lot of danger in our lives, our amygdala alarm system works overtime, and will be hyperactive and overreactive to the slightest detail. Our alarm system in the house would be easier to set off and harder to settle.

The amygdala has a storage cupboard called the hippocampus. The hippocampus stores memories, especially emotive ones. The more unhealed trauma we're holding, the more crammed our storage cupboard will be. Also, the more emotive a memory is, the more it gets in the way of our amygdala and its senses. This makes it harder for our alarm system to distinguish the difference between a past trauma and the present and so it begins to hold on to the traumatic memories, more than the pleasant or neutral ones.

This is why some people experience flashbacks. The amygdala alarm system notices a snippet of sensory information (a smell, sight, sound, taste or texture) and the hippocampus checks whether we can match it up with something in storage. When it pairs up with something traumatic, our alarm system goes into panic mode. For example, hearing a song that reminds us of an ex-partner can take us right back to our heartbreak in just a few seconds.

Now let's go upstairs, where we have the bedroom and relaxing bathtub, the more intimate spaces. It is the highest point in the house and where we go to rest, think, plan, feel and gain perspective. In the brain, this is known as the Pre-Frontal Cortex (PFC). This part is focused on feeling our emotions and making sense of them. The PFC is the calmest part of our mind, where we are able to soothe by regulating our feelings, control our impulses and empathize with ourselves and others. It's also the part of our brain which can reflect and make sense of things, as well as naming our feelings. It's the place where we have our 'eureka' moments. It is where we have our deepest and more reflective thoughts. Like those intimate late-night chats with a friend after a night out. All of that happens in the PFC.

In contrast to our amygdala alarm system, the PFC takes the longest to develop. It doesn't reach full development until the age of 25. This is why it's easy for us to look back on the actions of our younger selves with slight embarrassment, because once we hit our mid-twenties our brain has the reflective capacity to gain hindsight. This also means that upstairs is the least visited room in our brains and we don't naturally allocate much mental space to these rooms. They can be easily forgotten, especially in the middle of chaos or trauma. Therefore, it takes a lot of practice and persistence to make them more familiar.

Just like most houses, our brain often takes a bottom-up approach. This means we can't go upstairs without starting downstairs first. We also can't be upstairs and downstairs at the same time. So usually, information is checked out downstairs first by the alarm system before it's given permission to continue upstairs for deeper thought and reflection.

I tell my clients to imagine their brains as a house party when they're triggered. Downstairs will be loud and chaotic, and can leave us feeling anxious or agitated. The best thing we can do is to find a quiet room upstairs where we can bring ourselves back to balance again.

Grace, a client of mine had a panic attack one day whilst walking in a busy neighbourhood with her partner. She said it had happened very suddenly and for 'no reason at all'. We gently backtracked to what happened that day and I asked Grace what sights, sounds and smells she remembered.

A detail that stood out to me was that she recalled a strong smell of alcohol as they walked past a group of men drinking on the pavement. I asked if the smell of alcohol could be a trigger for her and if she had any difficult memories connected with it. Grace went silent for a moment, before I saw the recognition on her face. She shared how she connected the smell of alcohol with difficult memories from her childhood, as her abuser would often be heavily drunk when close to her.

Together we discovered that the smell of alcohol coupled with the fear of walking past a group of drunk men had triggered her alarm system to believe she was in danger again, sending a rush of adrenaline and cortisol that sent her body into a panic attack. She had been trapped in her downstairs brain, and unable to reflect that she was actually safe and in good company.

We worked together to recognize more of her triggers, things that told her brain that she wasn't safe. We also looked at things that helped her feel safe, to regulate her back to a calm state. By doing this, she could calm her downstairs brain in moments of panic and anxiety.

Just like it happened for Grace, *knowing* that we're safe isn't the same as *feeling* safe. We can consciously know that we are in a safe place, with safe company or in a safe part of our lives, but we can still feel unsafe or triggered. When our brain relies on our five senses to scan for danger, it can throw us back into the trauma of a difficult memory that we haven't yet healed from. Even if our brain isn't always consciously aware, our body remembers what triggers us. But our triggers don't have to torment us forever.

So let me reassure you: just like a house, your brain can be changed and renovated. Though your early or traumatic experiences leave a mark on how it functions, your brain is adaptive enough to change when you have new experiences. This is called plasticity. Essentially, the brain adapts to protect you from trauma, but it can also adapt to heal you through trauma. Like I said, your brain is a beautiful thing.

The key to heal through our trauma is to build and decorate the stairs. We need to find more ways to move from our downstairs brain to our upstairs brain. One way to do this is to discover ways to soothe our alarm system, by letting it know that we are safe in the here and now. When we do this, we soothe the chaos of our reactive downstairs brain, allowing us access to the more complex functions of our brain. This gives us the ability to reflect and remember the most important thing: we are now safe.

Here's an exercise to help you with that:

Exercise: Triggers and Glimmers

Our amygdala alarm system is in charge of working out
how safe we are by using our senses. If we see, smell, taste,
hear or feel something is **not safe**, we will feel **fear**. These
are called **Trauma Triggers**.

But the opposite is also possible. When we see, smell,
taste, hear or feel something is **safe**, we feel **comfort** and
love. Trauma expert Deb Dana calls these **Glimmers**.
Glimmers remind us that we are safe, by connecting
us to a comforting memory or the safety of the present
moment. For example, the taste and warmth of a cup
of hot cocoa might bring us back to reality after being
triggered.

Our alarm system is there to protect us, so we don't
want to turn it off. However, we do want to stop it from
overreacting. We can use our senses to reset our alarm
system whenever we need to. By engaging with things
that help us feel safe, we trick our brain and our nervous
system into calming down and returning to the present
moment.

Here's your invitation to create a list of your trauma
triggers and glimmers. Think about people, places and
things that can set off or calm your amygdala alarm
system. And don't forget to share this list with your loved
ones so they know how to take care of you when you need
it.

	Triggers = Danger	Glimmers = Safety
Smells		
Sounds		
Sights/Colours		
Tastes		
Textures/Touch		
Physical Sensations		
Places		
People/ Characteristics		

Survival mode

Trauma makes us do funny things. It gives some of us a stronger sense of humour because we've had to learn to laugh through the pain. Some of us become advocates, standing up for others in the ways we wish someone would have stood up for us. Whether we recognize it or not, these are trauma responses which become part of the fabric of our lives.

Because life moves quickly, many people have little awareness of the traumas that they might be carrying with them. Just like a heavy backpack, even if we forget what we're carrying, our body still feels the weight of it. Thanks to our alarm system and storage cupboard, the body remembers trauma even when we're not consciously aware of it. When we have unresolved trauma, our brain continues to alert our body to triggers.

Trauma can control the ways that we behave. I call this survival mode, where we have to keep on keeping on with unresolved trauma. Our brain then recruits trauma responses to protect us from further pain. These trauma responses are:

Fight – Our alarm system signals for the body to release adrenaline in preparation to fight or attack our trigger. Example: Bruce Banner turns into the Hulk to fight villains.

Flight – Our alarm system signals for the body to release adrenaline in order to run away or hide from our trigger. Example: in *The Lion King*, Simba runs away when his father dies.

Fawn – Our alarm system remains hypervigilant in order for us to read and cater to the needs of other people. Example: in the film *The Joker*, the main character learns to laugh through his pain.

Freeze – Our alarm system signals for our body to shut down and be immobile to avoid further danger and numb pain. Example: Tracy Beaker spends her time creating extravagant daydreams to deal with being in a foster home.

	FIGHT	FLIGHT	FAWN	FREEZE
PURPOSE	To protect or fight back	To avoid and run to safety	To appease and reduce conflict	To numb and shut down
THE BODY	Increased heart rate and breathing, muscles tensed, alert	Increased heart rate and breathing, muscles tremble, agitated and fidgety	Hypervigilant, looking outwards to the body language of others	Decreased heart rate and breathing, muscles relax, alert
Examples include:	Irritability, rage, aggression, pushing people away, over-controlling behaviour	Overworking, use of alcohol, drugs or sex to avoid feelings, overthinking	Using humour, poor boundaries, masking, hypervigilance to the needs of others	Dissociation, day-dreaming, binge-watching, escapism, brain fog

Trauma responses help to protect us at the time of our trauma and when we are triggered. However, eventually these survival methods no longer serve us. When this happens, they can turn into traits like:

- Toxic shame
- Self-sabotage
- Addiction
- Reactive decision-making
- Self-destruction
- Poor or rigid boundaries
- People-pleasing behaviours
- Avoiding sex or using sex to distract ourselves
- Chasing chaos

- Fear of intimacy
- Self-neglect
- Rationalizing trauma

In the therapy room, I often say how triggers are a sign that we are ready. We are ready to start looking deeper at what happened to us. The body is literally sending us a signal that something isn't right and we need to give it some TLC. Our triggers can be our teachers, teaching us where the pain is.

Our superpower is our ability to reverse-engineer what happened in the moment. When our body hypes up into fight-or-flight mode, we can learn to slow down and regulate our body back to safety and reflection. And when our body slows down into freeze, we can find ways to warm up and energize our body back to safety and connection. As for fawn, we will come back to that later, when we speak about boundaries. When we feel ready and safe, our PFC starts to do the maths of understanding what buttons were pushed in our trauma brain. The more we do this, the more we gain autonomy over our trauma.

Contagious trauma

What about when we can't pinpoint a trauma? Or what about when the trauma doesn't belong to us at all? And what about when trauma feels contagious?

Like a bowling ball thrown at pins, trauma can have a knock-on effect by vicariously traumatizing those who are connected to a trauma survivor. This can happen through intergenerational trauma and secondary trauma.

Intergenerational trauma

Intergenerational trauma, or trans-generational trauma, describes the way that trauma can be passed down from generation to generation. It starts with a trauma happening within a specific generation, which impacts a family, collective or intersectional group of people. A generational trauma can happen on a personal, interpersonal or group level. The way that the wounded group survives and adapts to trauma impacts each generation that comes afterwards. This was first noticed many years after the Holocaust, when it was recorded that children of Holocaust survivors were 300 per cent more likely to have negative mental health than their grandparents, despite being born two generations after the Holocaust period. Other examples include:

- The colonialization and the intergenerational trauma of Black and Brown people.
- The AIDS crisis of the 1980s which led to a political and social discrimination against gay men, causing intergenerational trauma of queer people.
- In families with a history of physically or emotionally absent parents, where the lack of a positive role-model can lead to continued patterns.

One thing I love about Disney is how they make children's stories relevant for adults. My favourite example of intergenerational trauma comes from the awesome Disney film *Encanto*. If you haven't watched it, here is the excuse you were waiting for. And if you have watched it, yes, we can finally talk about Bruno.

The film centres around a Columbian family called the Madrigals. They happen to have various magical gifts which they are told were bestowed on them by a higher power in order to serve the community. In reality, the magical gifts came during an event of deep trauma. Generations prior, Abuela Alma, the grandmother of family had been forced to flee from her hometown with the rest of her community due to political violence. Her trauma continued as the community were attacked by bandits, leading Alma to witness the killing of her husband. It was from this moment that her pain and fear built up, leading her magical gifts to appear for the first time, which she used to protect her and the rest of the community. All of this happened whilst she was pregnant with triplets.

The trauma of this story is never spoken about with the younger generations of the family. Instead, she presents values of strength, servitude and toxic positivity which everyone in the family must uphold. We watch as the grandchildren feel the immense pressure that comes with fulfilling these impossible expectations, leading to anxiety, perfectionism and internalized shame. Just like Bruno, anyone who doesn't fit into these expectations is shamed, rejected and essentially scapegoated.

The film highlights a few things about generational and intergenerational trauma:

Trauma leaves a mark on our genetic make-up

Though our DNA sequence stays the same, the study of epigenetic processes shows how traumatic events can influence the way our genetic make-up expresses itself. In *Encanto*, it's likely that Alma always had the genetic ability to have a magical gift. However, the trauma she experienced is what activated these genes, leading future generations to inherit these genes already activated (i.e. they had magical gifts without having to experience direct trauma first).

Perinatal capacity is important

As we learned in an earlier chapter, the first few years of our life shapes our attachments and security. During that time, the traumas that a parent holds (including how *they* were parented) will influence their own emotional capacity. With Abuela Alma, we can imagine that she gave birth whilst grieving the love of her life and having a whole community looking to rely on her magical talents. This would have impacted her children and then *their* children.

We learn our survival mode from our parents

How we cope with stress and trauma is taught to us by our parents. As children, we pick up on the ways they cope (or don't cope) and adopt those as our own.

Inherited trauma responses can look like gifts

Often the ways our ancestors had to adapt to survive become glamorized as gifts or traits to be proud of. For example, many immigrant families, like in *Encanto*, uphold values about strength, hard work and serving the community, but then minimize the value of vulnerability, rest and self-care. This is because these were not accessible at the time of the generational trauma that occurred.

Being an intergenerational cycle-breaker is tough

Just like Bruno, trying to make changes to the intergenerational trauma system is hard and can come with judgement and resistance from others.

There are so many avenues by which trauma gets inherited. However, in the words of Kazu Haga, when we carry intergenerational trauma, we're also lucky enough to carry intergenerational wisdom. And so, when we heal ourselves, we also heal the next generation.

Exercise: Family Tree

Draw a family tree, thinking about the history of your family.

Reflect on any of the following:

What beliefs, values and life lessons were passed down through the generations and down to you?

What traumas might have been at the root of these?

> Are there any coping strategies or specific trauma
> responses that have travelled from the history of your
> family?
>
> What stories were passed down?
>
> What gifts were passed down to you?
>
> Were any of these from potential trauma?
>
> What familial/cultural beliefs or stigma stood in the way
> of your healing?
>
> What lessons of wisdom are you learning now that you'd
> like to pass on to the next generation?

Secondary trauma

Another way that trauma shows up indirectly is through secondary trauma. This type of trauma happens when we witness or hear about the trauma of someone else which then impacts our own trauma brain.

In May 2020, the world was changed by the murder of George Floyd, an African American man who was unjustly killed by the police. There was recorded footage of his death and resulting protests, which was circulated on social media again and again.

I remember feeling numb and vulnerable that week. I distanced myself from friends and found myself crying alone. My trauma brain was triggered and I went into freeze response. I never knew George Floyd and I live a thousand miles from America but there was an undeniable closeness that I felt to mourning him. Viewing how his life was taken felt too close to home for me. Each time I saw the footage, I would imagine the same thing happening to one of my Black male family members or my partner. It was a vivid reminder that, as a Black woman, I was not safe and nor was my tribe. To know that my safety could be taken away because of my skin colour triggered secondary trauma. Someone else's suffering provoked my own.

This is just one example of how secondary trauma can travel thousands of miles and still have a physical and emotional impact. Groups of people who are most prone to secondary trauma include:

- First responders, doctors and nurses
- Therapists, counsellors, mental-health phone-line operators
- Teachers
- Those from a marginalized group
- Those who are supporting a loved one with trauma.

When secondary trauma shows up, it often looks like fatigue. We might feel emotionally depleted, numb or dissociating. Our 'freeze' trauma response is triggered because we have overfilled our emotional capacity. When this happens we need:

Boundaries: Set clear boundaries about how much help you can support someone with. As human beings, we have a capacity that we need to keep adjusting and listening to.

Inner-child love: When you're triggered, a helpful thing to do is give yourself nurture. You may be feeling as though your own needs have been neglected and so it's time to attend to these again.

Get support: Whether you are a therapist, teacher or friend, it's important that you have your own space for emotional support too. Lean into getting support from other friendships, mentors or supervision.

Movement is medicine

Our body remembers trauma. Even when we're unaware of it, it shows up in physical ways. We might experience headaches, stomach aches, jumpiness or chronic pain. Our mind might feel like we're 'over it', but our body doesn't yet know or realize that we are in fact safe again. This is because of the cortisol (stress hormone) which is running through our body before and after trauma. It needs to dissipate, and if it doesn't, it can give us some nasty and difficult symptoms. So as much as we need to heal emotional trauma, we also have to heal it somatically within the body and nervous system too.

One way of doing this is through movement. Movement practices like dance and yoga help to slow down our nervous system and move it into rest and digest mode, through deep breathing and fluid movement. I spoke with Imogen Ivy, a curve model and body-positivity influencer who shared with me her own experiences with trauma and healing somatically.

> *For over six years, I was misdiagnosed and mistreated for a physical illness that I didn't have. It made me incredibly sick in many ways, including my organs. I was unlucky, overlooked and slipped through the cracks. And though I'm now in good health, it left me with medical PTSD. My PTSD symptoms included anxiety, repetitive thoughts, flashbacks and nightmares.*
>
> *Nine months in, I had the sudden urge to want to move my body. I realized that movement is a privilege. I would just dance in my knickers in my living room. I didn't care what I looked like, it made me feel alive. I started to notice a lot of emotion coming up.*
>
> *Some days I cried and it felt like a release. It felt good so I decided to try moving my body continuously for one minute through fluid movements. I started to call it 'flowing' and it felt like my body was doing the talking. With time, just like meditation, the noises in my head stopped and eventually became blank.*

I was releasing my trauma through movement that was being stored within my limbs. My body remembered my trauma more than my brain had. This helped me to regain my memory, but I luckily had flowing to support me along that journey as well. Being curious, listening to and experimenting with my body has now led me to live a PTSD-free lifestyle. My PTSD no longer rules over me. I feel free and it all started from dancing in my living room in my knickers!

To someone struggling with trauma or PTSD, I would say: new chapters happen, so write them. You are not your trauma. You cannot change what's happened to you, but you can dictate the future. Trauma is like a backpack. You will never be able to take it off completely, but you sure can lighten that load. I don't feel my backpack any more. It will always be there but it doesn't weigh me down any more. Take your power back.

Movement is medicine for our healing. Alongside doing the internal work of healing our mind, we can't forget to give time and space to our body. Allowing your body to step out of the stuckness of a triggered nervous system will bring you closer to the healing you always needed.

Turning wounds into wisdom

Trauma shows up in almost every fiction book, film or television series that we watch. You'll know this if you're a DC fan, as every DC superhero or supervillain has a history of trauma that shapes their story – the origin story. Batman witnessed the murder of his parents and was left an orphan. Wade Wilson is diagnosed with terminal cancer before he becomes Deadpool. And my personal favourite, Harley Quinn, a psychiatrist, falls into a toxic, co-dependent relationship with her patient, aka The Joker, transforming her into his doting sidekick.

The assumption here is that normal people become superheroes (or supervillains) after their trauma. It transforms them into something powerful, yet it doesn't fully show the pain of recovery. As a society, we tend to put this expectation on to real life people experiencing real-life trauma. To soldier on and get on with things. To become superhuman. I once worked with an 18-year-old girl who had experienced a sexual trauma the year before. She was studying for her A levels and though her teachers were supportive, they were also really pissing her off. They would say that she was 'such a survivor' and an 'inspiration' in an attempt to encourage her and remind her of her strength. She told me how it made her freeze up every time she heard it and how it perpetuated the idea that she was never allowed to say when she was feeling vulnerable and in need of help. The therapy space was the only place where she had permission to take off her armour and let go of the expectation to be strong.

The truth is, healing has nothing to do with being strong. Strength is overrated. Healing is not straightforward or single-layered. An image I share with my clients is that healing from trauma is like a spiral staircase. We go around to the same point that we've been to before, but at a higher level. Our healing doesn't end, it evolves. Instead, resilience and reflection are our superpowers.

Good healing habits

Learning how to ditch shame and lean into self-compassion is one of the most important skills to learn when healing. It defines how we write the rest of our story and make sense of what happened.

Healing through ourselves

Just like a physical wound, recovery from a trauma wound takes a lot of time, patience and TLC. When it comes to healing, there are a few techniques that we can make use of. These get stronger the more that we practise them. Things to try:

- Journaling
- Reading books (like this) which help you understand and talk about trauma
- Finding helpful social-media content
- Creativity like painting or drawing what you feel.

Healing through our bodies

As Imogen beautifully taught us, movement is medicine. Healing through our bodies can be done by activating our parasympathetic nervous system, which is in charge of rest, recovery and restoration. Things to try:

- Mindfulness or tapping exercises
- Yoga
- Dance
- Stretching parts that get tense when stressed/triggered
- Massage
- Singing in a group or choir
- Finding sensory glimmers.

Healing alongside others

Though people can cause our trauma, safe people can help us repair it. Many emotional wounds are so deep that we need people in our lives to help us heal. Telling our stories and discovering who we are now with people who are compassionate and trustworthy can make healing through trauma much smoother. Talking to people we love also activates our PFC and upstairs brain, so it's a win–win. Things to try:

- Share what happened with someone you trust
- Find affirming spaces
- Try therapy with a trauma-informed therapist
- If you feel stable and supported enough, help others.

Just as Michael Rosen says in one of his children's books, there may be obstacles on the way and they may feel scary. But the only way out is through.

Real Talk on Trauma

- Trauma is an emotional wound.
- There are Big T and Small T traumas, but both can have a big impact on us.
- Childhood trauma can take a toll on our development as children.
- In the brain, we have an alarm system which responds to actual, potential and past trauma.
- Trauma triggers are sensory information that tell us we are not safe.
- Trauma glimmers are sensory information that tell us we are loved.
- Our trauma responses protect us from further pain, but they can also turn into traits that no longer serve us. These are fight, flight, freeze and fawn.
- Trauma can be passed down from generation to generation or from witnessing someone's experience. But healing can also be passed down and contagious.
- Resilience and reflection are our superpowers.
- The only way out is through.

6

What Holds Us Back

The more we've been hurt, the stronger our armour.

We've talked about how our brain deals with trauma, but what about our mind and soul? The ripple effect that trauma has on who we become is somewhat inevitable, but when bad shit happens, we shift and adapt. We put our armour on and build new walls to protect ourselves and to become bulletproof from any further pain. But the thing is, when we do this we also lock ourselves in with the pain and trauma that we're already carrying.

We pick up clever ways to shield ourselves, something that therapists call 'defences'. And though these defences are designed to keep us safe from pain, they also keep us at arm's length from all things vulnerable: they end up being defences against our own healing and self-love. Defences are antithetical to our growth and stand in the way of us being our most authentic and real selves. So which do we choose? Protecting ourselves from future pain or opening ourselves up to heal?

Our Inner Batman

The saying often goes 'Fool me once, shame on you; fool me twice, shame on me'. None of us wants to be hurt in the same place twice. So when we have been hit by trauma or pain, we adapt ourselves to avoid being hit again. Trauma makes us want to protect ourselves. And the part of us that most wants that protection is our ego.

Ego isn't always about arrogance, as most people assume. Our ego is one part of our mind and its main role is self-preservation. Our ego protects us from emotional pain like shame, guilt and betrayal. And the more we have been hurt, the stronger the armour of our ego becomes. On an unconscious level, our ego is constantly figuring out what we need to do to keep us safe, strong and respectable. Naturally, we all lead with our ego. It's like the armour and shield that a soldier might wear which brings them a sense of control and protection. But eventually we need to reassure ourselves that we can lower our shield and allow ourselves to be fully seen without it.

We can think of defences like weapons of war that we use against vulnerability. We use them to attempt to feel stronger, tougher or more indestructible. And though it might give us moments of feeling those things, the only thing that will make us stronger and more resilient is learning how to get comfortable with our vulnerability. Defences make us defensive. Two countries at war have the choice to put up their defences and release their cannons. But the only thing that will actually solve the conflict and stop the war is if they allow themselves to be vulnerable enough to see each other eye to eye. It's only then that they can discuss how to resolve the conflict and how to move forward in harmony. The same applies to us: we have a choice to keep our walls up or to give permission for harmony within ourselves.

There are lots of different defensive weapons that we use. We have some weapons that attack our own vulnerability. Sigmund Freud described a few of these defences many years ago. Here are some relatable ones:

DEFENCE	WHEN OUR EGO IS . . .	EXAMPLE
Denial	Refusing to be aware of something painful	This is not happening. I don't want to know.
Repression	Pushing difficult experiences out of our memory	Oh, really? I can't remember that.
Projection	Seeing ourselves in other people	I'm not the problem. You're the problem.
Regression	Acting like a younger version of ourselves	Why are you picking on me?
Humour	Covering difficult feelings with comedy or laughter	I hate my life, haha, just kidding.
Displacement	Shifting our emotions to the wrong person	I'm not angry at you, I'm angry at the situation.
Intellectualization	Using intellect to explain a situation instead of feeling it	Let's analyse this without getting emotional.
Rationalization	Justifying to explain a situation instead of feeling it	I'm not crying. It's my allergies.

Real Talk Moment:

- *Do you recognize yourself in these defences?*
- *Don't be too hard on yourself if you do, as we all experience them. Take note of which defences feel familiar and when.*
- *What could you give yourself in that moment instead of using a defence?*

As Carl Jung said, what we resist persists. Whatever truth we try to bash away using our defences is only temporary. The truth that we're frightened of will find other ways to come back to us, no matter how many defences we have in place. Our defences are the aftermath of existing within survival mode. The more we've been hurt, the stronger our armour.

When we've experienced trauma, grief or pain, we can often go into a place of blaming ourselves, especially if we're coming from childhood trauma. Our inner child can't work out why someone would let us down the way that they did. Taking the blame or accountability as a result gives us an illusion of control – it's a defence. And if there's one thing our ego loves, it's control. Control is how we protect ourselves from being vulnerable. Our ego says, *'Why me? What is it about me that is so unlovable or so inadequate that I get treated this way? Well, I'm never letting that happen again, so let me change myself to prevent anyone doing me wrong ever again.'* So even if it hurts to blame ourselves, taking accountability means we have control over fixing the problem and don't need to tap into the vulnerability of finding the root cause of these feelings.

Jungian analyst and clinical psychologist Donald Kalsched calls this our Self-Care system. This shouldn't be confused with what we call self-care in wider terms, aka the ways that we look after our wellbeing. This self-care system is more about the ways we momentarily 'take care' of our selves by doing two things. The first thing that happens is that we create a tough part, and this part of us acts as our protector. We create our bodyguard, our tough shell, our protector. This part of us wants to be both respected and admired, is intolerant of shame or pain and builds a wall around itself. The second thing that our self-protection system does is to lock our vulnerable, traumatized parts away for no one to see. This part is the wounded part of us. This 'locking away' affects our inner child, who wants to be held, loved and comforted but is also scared of shame and disappointment. Because it is so fiercely protected by the tougher parts, it is starved of the emotional connection that it needs. My favourite description comes from David Taransaud, a child psychotherapeutic counsellor, who says it's as if our tough parts take our vulnerable parts hostage. Our hostage taker is the only part of us that we let most people meet.

Let me demonstrate this through the story of Bruce Wayne, aka Batman. In the Batman comics, Little Bruce Wayne is just a child when he witnesses both his parents murdered at the hands of a mugger. The death of a parent is one of the most painful traumas that a child can go through, let alone both parents. Bruce finds himself orphaned with no other relatives to take him in, other than his loyal butler, Alfred, The trauma and vulnerability that had suddenly entered his life was so unbearable. So young Bruce locks away that part of him, the little orphan boy traumatized from losing his parents. Instead he quickly matures and hardens to become Batman, declaring that he will avenge their deaths by fighting injustice and fighting off the criminals of Gotham City. He devotes himself to intense physical and intellectual training. The little orphan boy is his vulnerable self and Batman is his protective self.

Becoming our protective self gives us temporary comfort. For Bruce Wayne, it gave him control (*This will never happen again because I'll get rid of all the criminals in town*). It gave him distraction from his emotional pain (*I have a purpose and I'm too busy to grieve*). It gave him protection (*Anyone who comes for me will lose the fight*). But it also kept him in a loop of his own trauma. As we know from the Batman comics and films, bad guys never stop walking the streets of Gotham City, so his quest is tireless. Not only that, but it stands in the way of him living his life fully and fearlessly. It hinders his capacity for meaningful friendships, relationships and self-love. And let's not forget that he could never be his authentic self in case his true identity is discovered.

This is the reason why we sometimes hold on to our traumas

aggressively. Instead of moving towards the softness of healing, we might fear the unknown of who we are behind our false, protective identity. Even Christian Bale hinted at this once in an interview about his role as Batman, describing how Bruce wants to maintain the anger that fuels the feeling of injustice that makes him Batman. But all of the energy we spend being driven by our trauma is lost energy for getting to know who we really are.

The problem with this self-care system is it throws us off the course of our natural path of growth. When we lock up the vulnerable part or our inner child like Bruce did, that part of us becomes sheltered and without healing. Even though Bruce grew into an adult who became Batman, he was very much still a little boy being directed by his little-boy pain. His wounds cut deep but he refused to attend to them, and this can also happen to us when we lock up our vulnerable parts. The downside of this is that we mature too quickly, missing out on vital stages that we need for trauma healing and growing into healthy human beings living our best lives. Bruce struggles to trust others or have intimate relationships because of this.

If you've experienced trauma, it's likely that you have had your own Inner Batman moment. Whilst you might not necessarily be a vigilante fighting the criminals of your local town at night, it may have shown up in different ways:

Hyper-independence

A common way that our Inner Batman shows up is through hyper-independence. If we didn't feel held as children by our caregivers or environment, we learn to hold ourselves. Being betrayed, let down or hurt by loved ones teaches us that we cannot trust people, we can only trust ourselves. So we might become over-independent, self-reliant and self-sufficient by promising to only stand on our own two feet and without help or support. We learn to take on more than we can handle and have no idea how to ask for help and support. For the most part, Batman's only road to support is his butler whose help he often actually rejects. Alfred is always telling Batman to slow down and be kinder to himself, but the advice is ignored. Being dependent on only ourselves doesn't allow us to form new, trustworthy relationships or to build our own social skills. As human beings, we were not born to exist in isolation. Our brains are built to thrive in a supportive community.

Saviour/Rescuer

Going through trauma or loss makes us hypervigilant to the trauma and loss of other people, and we might have a belief that we need to rescue them from their own pain. In reality, we're trying to rescue the vulnerable part of us, our Little Us, over and over again by being the saviour to other people. This is problematic as we might believe we are the *only* ones who can save the people around us. Being the rescuer means that we are attracted to vulnerability in other people but are unable to attend to our own. And whilst it is a sign of our capacity for empathy, being a saviour might mean that we see people as projects that we need to fix and change. And just like Batman, dedicating our lives to being the hero for other people can lead to burnout, resentment and a lack of life fulfilment.

Victim mode

Victimhood might sound a little out of place since we're talking about the negative impacts of shutting away our vulnerable parts, but hear me out. Whilst we can be valid victims or survivors of trauma, a victim mentality is different since it is a coping strategy that doesn't serve us. It works by applying the pain that we felt from trauma to the rest of our ongoing narrative, so we *expect* to be victimized in all situations. For Bruce Wayne, his victimhood showed up in how he holds lifetime grudges and his ruminating thoughts of Gotham as a bad city. This could also look like blaming others and making excuses for our own behaviour, inability to reflect and take personal responsibility, unable to empathize or connect with other people's pain and mistrust in others. It also includes purposely not connecting with things that we know would make us feel better, like therapy or self-care activities. We purposely choose to not engage with self-love or healing. We pick up a learned helplessness, where we believe that life is always unfair and there's nothing we can do about it. By placing ourselves in the role of victim, we get to avoid real vulnerability, accountability and doing the work needed to heal.

Identification with the aggressor

Have you heard the saying 'hurt people hurt people'? Well this is what Anna Freud, Freud's daughter, called Identification with the Aggressor. The idea is that when we've experienced something that we haven't healed from, we project it onto other people. Bruce Wayne's parents were hurt by criminals and he projects this by becoming a vigilante who hurts criminals. He learns to identify with the actions of the people who caused his pain, the aggressors. Rather than healing his pain, he re-enacts it on other people, justified by his moral code. For the everyday person, this would look more like treating our spouse or children the way that our parents treated us. Or feeling shamed by a colleague at work and then going home to shame our partner in a similar way. Or a child who is bullied at home becomes the playground bully at school. This happens because of the temporary relief to feel powerful and in control, and to experience being on the other side of our pain by inflicting it. This is problematic since it creates a chain of trauma that is being passed on from one person to the next.

In therapy, most people will bring along their Batman selves long before they show me their Bruce Wayne. They may unconsciously hide behind things like their jobs, successes or their independence because they have become the personality of their Inner Batman. These are the things that bring us control, respect and admiration, and so are naturally easier for our ego to talk about. In the same way, most people will express tougher feelings of anger, frustration and annoyance before they show more vulnerable feelings like shame, sadness and longing. It may be months or years before they allow themselves to meet their Bruce Wayne. They are holding on to the story that they need to be strong, resilient and bulletproof.

We can't rush the work of exposing our own Batman. Just like any other hostage situation, we have to go into a hostage negotiation with care and patience. We talk to the hostage taker and gain their trust, before asking if we can see whether the vulnerable hostage is doing OK. Nor do we tell the hostage taker to stop being a hostage taker, because they're there for a reason, right? Instead, we need to find out what is their 'why' and 'how', so we can offer them another way to get what they need.

As Pema Chödrön says, we need to let our hearts break and drop the story. This means letting go of the expectations we put on ourselves of how we need to be, especially after trauma. Because the reality is, all you need to be is yourself. The more you lean into softness and vulnerability, the closer you step into your healing self, instead of your protective self.

Lean into the cringe

One of my favourite things to tell my clients is to *lean into the cringe*. Cringe describes a mixture of awkwardness, embarrassment and disgust. We might cringe when we see a couple showing public displays of affection. Or when we hear someone talk about their journey of self-love. Hell, you may even have cringed at pages in this book so far. But my beliefs about cringing is that we cringe at the things that we deeply need. Underneath the awkwardness, embarrassment and disgust exists a vulnerable part of us wanting the very thing that we cringe at. Fear makes us throw disgust on it, because how scary would it be to finally have our needs met, especially after trauma and pain? Think back to the last time *you* cringed. What unmet need was sitting underneath that awkwardness? Cringing happens when it feels too vulnerable to receive the goodness that we always deserved.

So, lean into the cringe. Let it soften your stomach and shift your armour. Just because that goodness was withheld from you at some point in your life, it doesn't mean that you don't or didn't deserve it. It's OK to receive it. It's also OK to admire it when we see it outside ourselves. Open your arms to the things that feel unfamiliar and vulnerable but also good and nurturing. Your protective self has done an awesome job of shielding you, but now it's time to open yourself up to nurture. Pass the mic to your Little Bruce Wayne so they can cut straight to the truth of what they need and want from you here on.

Exercise: Your Inner Batman

Take a moment to think about your inner Batman. Try to imagine what they would look like and be like. You may even want to draw them.

What weapons against vulnerability do they use and why?

What story are they holding on to about who you need to be?

What would dropping the story be like for you? What would you gain? What would you lose?

What have you been cringing at that you need to lean in to?

Saying hello to your shadow

As much as we might not be able to bear our feelings after trauma as individuals, the world that we live in doesn't know how to either. Big feelings don't have many places to go in this very big world. Toxic positivity is in the air, batting away anything awkward or emotional. And cancel culture has become a way to cut off from complicated and difficult conflict. So even though we all need softness and comfort after trauma, most of us will have to work hard to receive it because of how phobic the world is about vulnerable emotions. This gives us another reason to adapt ourselves and to hide our trauma.

In chapter 1, we spoke about the true self and false self. These are versions of ourselves that we all have, with or without trauma. The false self is the version of ourselves that we wear when we are navigating the outside world, and its expectations and needs. Our true self is our most genuine and real self sitting underneath, which ideally will have lots of safe spaces where it can exist and grow. These are the moments when big, strong Batman can feel safe enough to take a tea break from their shift and let Little Bruce Wayne out to play. It's the tender moments when we feel secure and in good company and can put down our façade and be our vulnerable, soft self again. Can you relate to those tender moments?

Because of how fearful culture is about vulnerability and trauma, these tender moments can be devastatingly rare. Not everyone around us knows how to deal with us when we're vulnerable. And this is especially the case if they've become so used to our tough exterior that meeting our softer layers might make them feel uncomfortable. As a society, we haven't been given the language to bridge the gap between the two parts of us. And that isn't your fault, it is just one of the ways that culture can let us down.

If we don't have any welcome spaces to bring up our vulnerability or our messy bits, we shut those bits down within us even more. We adapt ourselves to accommodate to the needs of everyone else. We strive to appear robust and resilient so as not to upset others with our messy feelings. We shape ourselves to fit this narrative. We are strong. We are kind. We are polite. We are composed. But what about all of the things that we *shouldn't* be? Where do those bits go? Let me introduce you to your Shadow.

We all have a darker side of our personality called our shadow. If our mind was a house, our shadow would be the basement, cellar or attic. It's the place where we hide all the difficult, ugly, awkward, uncomfortable, guilty, shameful crap in our unconscious. Carl Jung said that our shadow is the most 'guilt-laden' part of our personality. All of the things that we don't want anyone to see or know about is stored in this part of our psyche. It is made up of all the parts of us that we don't want to acknowledge. These secrets about us become so repressed that they become hidden from others but also hidden from ourselves.

Our shadow is moulded by social judgement and expectation. Everything we banish to our shadow is because society makes us see it as bad. As we'll see in chapter 7, we internalize an inner critic who tells us what we should do and who we should be. If our inner critic tells us who we should be, our shadow mops up everything that we believe we *shouldn't* be. And so we perceive these things as bad or unacceptable and banish them to the shadow of ourselves so that we no longer have to deal with it. We attach shame to personality traits that aren't acceptable for our age, gender, ethnicity, religion or family values. Our shadow knows a lot of our childhood wounds, and many things in our shadow got there because we were once told off or shamed for them as children. So we unconsciously vowed to shut it down and never be like that again. These secrets about us are out of sight, but never out of mind.

One of the things that used to make up my shadow was anger. Starting from childhood, I learned to hide my anger through smiling and politeness. The mantra 'kill them with kindness' was how I dealt with anger, and so I hardly ever expressed it. Being a Black girl in a white-dominated country, I learned to fear being the 'angry Black woman' trope that society puts upon people of colour showing anger. Society wrongly tells us that women are not allowed to be angry. It also wrongly tells us that Black people feeling anger equates to danger to society. Even if my anger was just, being the 'angry Black girl' would lead me to be feared, judged, shamed and for my feelings to be given an identity based on racist, misogynoir projections. So into the basement my anger went, until I was ready to face it in my own journey. For me, reading books like *Women Who Run With Wolves* helped me to reclaim the fiercer parts of my personality, including my right to anger.

> **Real Talk Moment:**
> - *Take a moment to think about what things were banished in your childhood or from wider society?*
> - *What were you told not to do, be, act?*
> - *Do you still banish those things within yourself?*

Our shadow is our *alter ego*, who is allowed to be themselves but when nobody else is looking. If you've ever seen a Peter Pan film, you'll remember his shadow as his trickster sidekick, causing havoc wherever he and Peter went. He causes mischief when Peter's not looking, like dancing and cartwheeling on the walls. In one of the films, Peter becomes detached from his shadow and feels completely lost because of it. Like an abandoned friend in need of our acceptance and attention, our shadow longs to be taken care of. Yet the more we ignore our shadow self, the more they will play up and have control over us unconsciously.

Accessing your shadow self

Believe it or not, there is so much beauty within our shadow selves. The parts of us that are cast aside are usually the most unique bits of us. The creative, driven, assertive, soft, weird or quirky parts that we've cast off in order to blend in. We have to meet with our shadow so that we can reclaim them as our conscious self. The more separated we are from our shadow, the further we are from being real with ourselves. Shadow work is about reuniting with parts of our shadow. Like finding missing pieces of a puzzle, by reconnecting the parts of us that we once rejected, we give ourselves permission to be our whole true selves. As Maya Angelou says, if we are always trying to be normal, we will never know how amazing we could be.

During my training as a psychotherapist, I experienced some shadow work whilst at a residential workshop. Creativity is like a direct phone call to our shadow, and so through a creative exercise the facilitator guided us towards our shadow selves. We were asked to create a paper sculpture of any object, so I created a rose bud. We were then asked to name how we are similar to our object and how we are dissimilar from the object. Now, just for context, I need to add that I was a bit of a wallflower in my twenties. My ethnicity, gender, birth order and childhood experiences had shaped me to be considerate, measured and very shy. And for this reason, I named how roses love to be at the centre of attention when this was something I feared with all my soul. Roses take up space that I couldn't take up myself. The idea of being ostentatious made me cringe. But remember what I said earlier: cringing can be a sign of something we need.

We were then asked to create a character based on this quality and to embody them in role play. My stomach flipped. But I went with it and I created my character, Chanel. Chanel was a social-media influencer with thousands of followers and a stinky attitude. She loved to be in the limelight and would throw anyone under the bus to maintain it. Chanel was ostentatious.

And guess what? I *loved* being Chanel. My body and soul felt a freedom that they had never felt before, where I didn't have to hold back my personality. My true self wasn't having to keep its mask on. In role play, I could be as arrogant, self-centred and sassy as I wanted to be. Being Chanel was a free pass to my shadow and many of the things that I had told myself not to be. She gave me permission to explore and play with characteristics I had rejected. And how funny to realize that five years later I would become a so-called influencer on social media myself. And though I hopefully don't have the stinky attitude, giving myself permission to take up space and find value in what I have to say likely came from a nudge from the Chanel within me.

For the most part, our shadow is unconscious. But our mind will always find ways to reveal our shadow back to us. Creative exercises are a positive way of inviting our shadow out to play, but our shadow can creep out in other, less positive ways, in everyday life too.

Projection and envy

We've all had that moment when we've fiercely disliked someone for no damn reason. We can't always put our finger on why we dislike them, we just know that we want nothing to do with them. This often happens because there's a quality in that other person that reminds us of our own shadow. We *project* the parts of us that we *reject*. As Carl Jung said, everything that irritates us about other people gives us a better understanding of ourselves. Whatever we reject in ourselves casts a shadow where we can see it.

Villains

Have you ever noticed yourself feeling connected to the villain in a story? Every fictional story has a shadow in the shape of an evil villain. And the reason why we need and gravitate to them in a narrative is that they represent a piece of our own shadow, since we're naturally attracted and sometimes repelled by people who remind us of our own darker bits. At the end of this chapter, I've set out a creative exercise to help you get to know your shadow a little better. But before we get to that, let's try something . . .

Imagine that you're hosting a dinner party for your shadow self. It's time to plan your guest list, and you can invite absolutely anyone, as long as they are fictional villains or unlikeable characters. Think about your favourite baddies of all time. Voldemort? Cruella? Regina George? Write a list of who you would invite, why you would invite them and what this might say about your own shadow.

Alcohol or Fatigue

When we're conscious in the day, our shadow is in the waiting room, biding their time for their next moment to be seen. These moments tend to be when we let our guard down and our ego is most relaxed, like when we're physically tired or drinking alcohol. How many times have you said something that you didn't mean to say when your guard is down in these moments? When our ego is tired, drunk or bored, it gives our shadow an opportunity to show up without our permission. Which is one reason why we might feel regretful about what we said the night after a party. It's no surprise that we are most likely to reveal our secrets when we're under the influence of alcohol. Being under the influence forces us to let go of control, because our inner critic closes for business. Alcohol or fatigue invites our shadow to do the talking for us.

Exercise: Dreams

Another way that our shadow peeks through is when we're not conscious. In other words, in our dreams. Our dreams are love letters from our subconscious, telling us what's really going on. Whatever our shadow is carrying turns up as we sleep, finally having the permission to reveal itself.

Dreams contain symbols and a storyline that have a million different meanings and can be interpreted in a million different ways. They hint at our shadow trying to communicate with us. One interesting example is that dreams about poo and needing the toilet are often linked to shame and repression. These types of dreams often come up when we're in therapy and learning how to *no longer repress* our messy feelings and experiences.

It can be helpful to note our dreams when they happen, using a notebook next to our bed or a notes app on our phone. Here are some prompts for working out your dreams:
What happened in the dream? Write down as much as you can remember. Include symbols, people, what you felt during the dream and what you felt when you woke up.
Pick out symbols or metaphors that really stood out. What does that symbol mean to you personally? What does it represent in your life right now?
What is your shadow trying to communicate with you? What do they want?

If you get stuck, ask a friend to help think about your dream with you.

Exercise: 3–2–1 Shadow Work

Now you've learned that you have a shadow self, it's time to own and reclaim it. 3–2–1 shadow work is a technique created by Ken Wilber. There are three steps that have to be done in order. It's OK if this feels a little cringy, and it's expected since we're about to get a little closer to the parts of you that you find hard to connect with in the first place. We will start small and you can come back to this exercise again and again to face different parts of your shadow in stages.

1. Face it – A lot of the time when we have strong feelings like irritation or an infatuation with someone which we can't explain, our shadow is at play. Irritation or obsession can be a sign of envy coming from our shadow. We might be seeing something in someone else that we've had to reject within ourselves.

Think of a person that angers, irritates or frustrates you. Or it can be a person who you are a little bit obsessed with but can't work out why. This could be a person you know well, or someone you don't know in person at all. You might want to start with a fictional character from film, television or a book, if you're feeling awkward.

Whoever it is, hold them in mind for a moment. Think about what it is that causes such a powerful reaction for you.

Now – this is important – say it aloud or write it down in third-person, he/she/they language. Describe the attributes and qualities about them that tugs on those feelings for you.

What do they do? What do they represent? You might even link why that attribute specifically rubs you the wrong (or right) way. For example, 'This person irritates me because they take up too much space.' Remember this person will never see or hear this, so give yourself permission to let it out and say what you need to say.

2. Talk to it – In order to reconnect to the things that we previously shut ourselves down from, it's important that we start to look at them in a non-judgemental way. Every quality exists on a spectrum. For example, we might see someone as being selfish but another viewpoint is that they are taking care of their emotional and physical needs by having clear boundaries.

I'd like you to have a conversation with this person to find out what those things might be. Move on to using second person, 'you' language. Imagine having a conversation with this person. What would you want to say, know or ask them? Say it aloud or write it down. Try to find the good in what they do that annoys you. Some questions you might ask are:

What do you want with me?

What are you here to teach me?

What's the story behind that irritating thing you do?

What do you have that I want or need?

Let yourself imagine what their response would be for each of these questions. Your shadow has lots to say, so don't forget to make notes.

3. Be it – Now we're going to own it by moving into the first person, using 'I' statements. Put yourself in the shoes

of your shadow and speak from their position. Connect
with the qualities about them that annoy you or entice
you. Embody the qualities that you named in part 1 and
take what you need to learn from part 2. Try finishing the
following sentences:

I am . . .

I need . . .

I embrace how . . . . . I am

Starting a journey of healing and self-love through embracing
our shadow often means that we focus on the things that we love
about ourselves, because these bits are easier than looking at the
things we don't. As Paulo Coelho says, we only see love's light, not
its shadows. Our Inner Batman and our shadow are usually the
bits of us that we don't want to acknowledge as much as we should.

But here's my gentle reminder for all of us to give love and light
to our shadow parts, letting them know they're welcome to exist
within us once again. Healing is about accepting all parts of us, and
especially the parts that are sitting in pain and shame, sitting in
the shadows. By inviting them to exist with us in the light, we grow
closer to being our most authentic and whole selves. Self-love isn't
just about loving yourselves but also discovering the parts of you
still waiting to receive that love.

Embracing your shadow doesn't dim your shine . . . It elevates
it.

Real Talk on What Holds Us Back

- Our ego always wants to protect us from being hurt, especially if it's already happened before.
- Our ego has different mechanisms of defences like denial and humour.
- Our Inner Batman is the part of us that protects us and hides our vulnerability away to do this.
- But having our vulnerability locked away holds us back from healing and self-love.
- We have lots of different ways of protecting ourselves, whether it's by defence mechanisms or changing our character.
- Our shadow is the part of us where we hide all of our unlikeable parts.
- A big part of healing is accepting all of the parts of our shadow and allowing them to be seen again.

7

Self-Esteem

Imagine if we allowed ourselves to obsess
about what we loved about ourselves,
instead of what we disliked?

Self-esteem tells us how 'good enough' we feel. People who struggle with self-love do so because the judgement and expectations they have of themselves are so loud. It's like an annoying song playing on repeat in our heads that we can't help but sing along to. Self-criticism runs around in our mind and we sing along to its self-deprecating tune. It chips away at our self-esteem and stands in the way of our healing.

Personally, this chapter has been hands-down the hardest for me to write. Let's be honest, I was avoiding it like hell. Writing this book has brought up so many personal insecurities. *What if I'm not good enough? Who do I think I am to write a book? What if nobody likes what I have to say? What if nobody likes me? Maybe I should stick to my day job . . . Wait, am I even good enough at that?* Each doubt was like a chain reaction, bringing more insecurities to my attention. And doubt loves to multiply.

These fears were soul-crushing to listen to and exhausting to battle with. They led to many days spent on the couch avoiding my writing deadline and telling myself that I'm a terrible writer, terrible therapist and everything I touch turns terrible. When our self-esteem is low, everything we see about ourselves is through shit-tinted glasses. We only see the worst of ourselves, and it can feel hard to hold on to pride, hope and compassion. We become our own enemy.

You'll notice from my experience that a lot of my fearful thoughts were about the things I *couldn't* control: whether people would like me or my writing is none of my business. Not having control is something that we struggle with as human beings, but it's unavoidable. Our thoughts do whatever they can to keep us inside our comfort zone, where things can stay under our control.

Our Self-Esteem Tank

Too many of us believe that it's arrogant to know our own self-worth. But actually, we all need a little sprinkle of narcissism. Narcissism is often talked about as a toxic trait and nobody wants to be called narcissistic. Our fear of narcissism means that so many of us brush away compliments, shy away from the spotlight or cringe when we need to speak about our strengths. But a healthy amount of narcissism helps us to thrive.

Ahead of his time, psychologist Paul Federn was the first to say there could be healthy narcissism in 1929. He told us that healthy narcissism was about a sense of self-love and being realistic in understanding what we are capable of achieving. Healthy narcissism is about having a strong foundation of regard, respect and love for ourselves. It's about how we see ourselves in relation to other people. This allows us to be resilient in receiving criticism from others and seeing feedback as a gift instead of a threat. We can admire and empathize with others, and we can also admire and empathize with ourselves. The fine line is how we respect ourselves without disrespecting other people in the process. Love for self is good. But love for self whilst invalidating others is bad. And narcissism *is* a vital ingredient for self-love.

Our first experience of narcissism comes from the day we are born. When our parents pour their love into us, we feel that love for ourselves too. Having a parent who listened to our cries and empathetically attended to our needs as babies builds us to have healthy self-esteem. We learn *I'm OK and I'm good enough*. But if we had parents who weren't able to meet us with empathy and attunement as babies, we learn to look for our sense of self, value and regard in other places.

Self-esteem is how we value and see the entirety of who we are. If self-love is the way that we commit and show love to ourselves, self-esteem is the lens that we do this through.

Imagine self-esteem as a tank that needs filling. It needs to be filled with hope, compassion and self-belief. The fuller it is, the more we can feed into our selves, our dreams and our relationships in a healthy way. We can smile back at our reflection and say *Hey, I'm good, I'm worthy, I'm important, I'm a badass*. We have enough in our self-esteem tank to practise self-love and to fuel our healing process.

But when our tank is empty, we need to fill it and it can make us hungry for external validation. We see ourselves and think *I could be better, I'm not enough, I bring nothing to the table, if only this part of me was different*. The emptier our tank is, the more we look to other people to fill it for us. We start to act and be who we think we need to be to impress and lure others. We move away from self-love and move into self-abandonment instead by meeting other people's needs before we try to acknowledge our own.

We've all heard of the phrase 'stroking your ego', right? When we're children, grown-ups help to fill and fuel our self-esteem tank with something called psychological strokes. The term comes from Eric Berne, who created transactional analysis, a type of therapy that works with the ego. He describes strokes as the way we recognize and acknowledge each other. Strokes are breadcrumbs of communication that make up the cake of how people see and value us. They are metaphorical pats on our back. Some are good and reassuring, whilst others feel harsh or demeaning. We could receive verbal strokes ('You look good'), physical strokes (a wink or squeeze of the shoulder). We could also receive written strokes (Employee of the Month) or the amount of time someone gives us can also feel like a positive or negative stroke too ('Your boss wants to see you'). Salespeople are particularly well versed in the language of strokes. Starting a conversation with a compliment and positive affirmations is often a sure-start way to get someone to buy into a conversation.

Strokes can feed or deprive our self-esteem. Each of us thrives when we receive signs that we are loved, appreciated, recognized and of value. It gives us a dopamine hit and confirmation that we're on the right path. Without it, we become stroke hungry and then we direct our behaviour in order to receive the strokes we're craving. Negative strokes trigger our amygdala alarm system and our stress responses so that we don't feel secure within ourselves. When this happens, our internal tank needs to be replenished with positive strokes.

Positive Conditional Strokes	Positive Unconditional Strokes
Tells us that we did something good *e.g. Awesome job!*	Tells us that we are good *e.g. You're so awesome, I like you*
Negative Conditional Strokes	**Negative Unconditional Strokes**
Tells us that we did something bad *e.g. That's the wrong answer*	Tells us that we are bad *e.g. You're an idiot, Bad boy!*

Let's imagine twins growing up in the same home. We'll call them Adam and Eve. The twins grow up with different experiences of strokes. Adam grows up with positive strokes right from the start. He is told he is a 'good boy' and 'beautiful baby'. He also hears that he is good at things like art and football. Because of an abundance of conditional and unconditional positive strokes, Adam grows up to feel good enough. How do you think this would shape his dating life, his friendships and his work?

Eve has a different experience. She is labelled as the 'difficult' baby and a 'needy' child. She's also told that she could do better at art and isn't very good at football. Unless she gets positive strokes somewhere else in her life, Eve grows up to feel not good enough. How do you think this would shape her dating life, her friendships and her work?

Real Talk Moment:
- *Which experience did you have?*
- *What types of strokes did you receive growing up? Positive or negative? Conditional or unconditional?*
- *How full is your self-esteem tank now as a grown-up?*
- *What strokes do you find easy or difficult to receive now as an adult?*

For too many of us, confidence building wasn't granted to us as kids. In childhood, we're often put in our place whenever we try to assert ourselves. Up until very recent generations, we weren't allowed to speak out of turn in the classroom and speaking up to grown-ups might have meant we were seen as disrespecting our elders. This behaviour might have been seen as talking back rather than voicing our needs and what's important to us. So it's no wonder so many of us struggle with confidence and speaking up for ourselves, when this was potentially seen as bad behaviour when we were growing up. Being assertive and being our own advocate might have come with a hell of a lot of shame and pushback from our elders.

The ghosts of our critical past

We each have an inner voice which narrates what we're feeling, thinking and doing. Our inner voice develops in childhood. Have you ever heard a child talk to themselves while playing or carrying out a task? You'll notice that they have full-blown conversations and this self-talk allows them to speak out their ideas and thoughts. This is what we eventually learn to do internally. Our inner voice has lots to say and comes in different forms. One of them is our inner critic.

Our inner critic takes up a lot of space in our heads. This is the voice that holds the most opinion, judgement, perfectionism and frustration. It might say things like *I should have done x, I'm crap at x, Why didn't I . . .'* This voice acts to guide and evaluate our behaviour, so that we can grow and do better next time. But sometimes the voice of our inner critic is a mean one. And its meanness depends on our experiences. The more critical experiences or higher expectations we had growing up, the fiercer our inner critic will be. For a lot of us, our inner critic repeats the words of adult caregivers. How we were told off and disciplined as a child is how we criticize ourselves as adults. Criticism that came our way as children becomes stored and released as our inner critic. Having authoritarian parents, over-protective siblings, harsh teachers and experiences of bullying can become a cruel gang of inspiration for the voice of our inner critic. It's an internalized identification with the aggressor, which we spoke about in chapter 6. In this case, sticks and stones won't break our bones, but harsh words we internalize and repeat back to ourselves until we heal them.

Sometimes we might find our inner critic telling us things that we've actually already heard before. A friend of mine went backpacking around the world, something her parents didn't approve of. Whilst on her travels, my friend happened to miss one of her flights. Stuck in the airport overnight, she was upset and berated herself heavily. *What's wrong with me? I should have done this. I should have done that. I never should have come in the first place. This is so irresponsible of me.* She decided to call her parents in hope of some comfort and support. But when she explained to them what had happened, they both berated her. Not only did they criticize her during her time of need but they said the same words that she had already said to herself. *What's wrong with you? You should have done this. You shouldn't have done that. You never should have gone in the first place. This is so irresponsible of you.* Her conversation with her inner critic had been a dress rehearsal for her IRL critics. And the source? Being the eldest daughter, she was always expected to be 'the responsible one'. But no matter how much she tried, she was never responsible *enough* in their eyes. When we find ourselves berating ourselves like my friend did, it's important to ask the question: whose voice is this?

We all have what I call ghosts from our critical past. These are memories of people who made us feel 'not good enough' when we were younger. They either said or did something that made us feel ashamed, guilty or rejected. Wanting to protect us, our brain holds on to these memories and remind us of them when similar situations or feelings come up in adulthood. Even if the person is no longer in our lives, the internalized memory has a lasting effect. It becomes part of the aura of our inner critic.

To take away some of the power from our inner critic, we need to deal with the ghosts of our critical past. By recognizing the past memories attached to our inner critic, we can release the hold they have on us.

Exercise: Ghosts of Your Critical Past

Name a ghost from your critical past. They could be a
grown-up or peer from your childhood years who made you
feel not good enough.
Who and what happened?
What did they say or do that knocked your confidence?
How did you feel then? How do you feel now as you
remember it? What does it feel like in your body?
How does this ghost show up in your inner critic now?
What do they say?
What do you wish you could have said to the ghost of your
critical past at the time?
What things can you say to these ghosts when they revisit
you?

Navigating our inner critic can be like having a boxing match
with ourselves. In one corner of the ring is the part of ourselves that
wants to win, have joy and success. And then, in the other corner,
we have the side of us that is so terrified of failure that they're
willing to knock us down in one punch before we take the risk.

Our brain is a feedback loop, which means that it's always
comparing reality to expectation. It looks for what is missing
and not good enough, so that we can take action to fix it. An easy
example is our ideal room temperature. When we enter a room,
one of the things our brain does is to check if the room matches
our ideal body temperature. If it's too cold, we get a jumper or
make a comment about how cold it is. If it's too hot, we take off a
layer or fan ourselves, making a comment about how hot it is. This
is our brain evaluating ourselves. Our brains are more inclined to

ask *what is wrong* rather than *what is right*. Unfortunately, most of the time we don't even pay attention to when things *are* right, we just look for the next thing for our brain to fuss over. We evaluate ourselves from a place of *what did I not do?*

This means we tend to do much better at naming our weaknesses than our strengths. Does that feel familiar at all? I notice this a lot when friends, clients or I myself have to prepare for annual work reviews. We can often expect the worst and list hundreds of things that make us not good enough at our jobs this year. But when it comes to listing what we're good at, we instantly struggle or shy away. This is why gratitude journaling can be a great tool, because by focusing on the positives we are disrupting the negative feedback loop of criticism, disappointment and a need for constant self-improvement.

Our inner critic is also super-confusing for our nervous system. In chapter 5, we spoke about the amygdala alarm system and how, when triggered, it sets off a trauma response: fight, flight, fawn or freeze. Well, it can also be set off by our inner critic. If our inner bully is hardcore on us, then our own thoughts become a threat to us. Wild, huh? Our own thoughts are the predator that we need to escape from and so our brain is triggered in the same way. In response, we might fight (get angry and frustrated at ourselves for pissing off our inner critic), flight (fear, avoidance and procrastination), freeze (shame, dread and shutdown) or fawn (fake it until we make it but at a cost to our self-care). And each of these has their own physiological responses too, so our inner critic could lead us to heart flutters, panic attacks or spacing out from our own thoughts.

Our inner critic isn't necessarily always trying to bring us down. In fact, I'd argue that our inner critic actually cares about us so much that it becomes like an overprotective older sibling. In its own weird way, it wants the best for us, but only if that means avoiding the risk of rejection and embarrassment. So it tries to scare and persuade us out of stepping out of our comfort zone. Our inner critic believes that there are worse critics out there in the world. And though that could be true, there is nothing more damning than having a critic living in your head rent free.

Our inner critics are creatures of habit and they dislike change that sits outside of their control. And so the more we step out of our comfort zone, the louder our inner critic gets. This is why when we're in the process of healing from old wounds and breaking old patterns, our inner critic might have a lot to say about it. They will make us feel guilty for implementing the boundaries that we always needed and they will torment us when we decide to take up more space in being vulnerable with others. Our inner critic feels content when we stay in the lane that our past experiences put us in to begin with. Newness can feel unsafe for our nervous system and our amygdala alarm system will call our inner critic in to micro-manage the situation. Healing and growth isn't a priority for our inner critic, but familiarity is.

Real Talk Moment:

- *What does self-criticism look like for you?*
- *When does it show up most?*
- *Does it fill you with encouragement, love and self-belief? (Probably not. It's more likely that it fills you up with dread, guilt and shame, which eventually forces you into doing whatever you need to do. But it's not a joyful or easy journey.)*

Exercise: Externalizing Your Inner Critic

Even though our inner critic is the villain in our hero story, we can't banish them entirely. Up until this point, they've served a purpose in our lives. But we no longer need them taking up so much space. So it's time to create some separation between them and us.

So, give your inner critic a name. It can be absolutely any name you want. This is another example of externalization. By giving your inner critic a name, you're separating them from yourself and your other inner voices.

When you notice your inner critic piping up, practise challenging them back. There might be some moments where you need to say 'Shut it, Bob' or to have a gentler approach of 'Hey, Bob, I see what you're trying to do here. But I don't need you right now, I've got this.' If he's being particularly tough, ask him to show the receipts and proof of his negative claims against you.

Since you no longer need Bob to be your inner critic, give them a new job title. For example, could they be a risk assessor or cheerleader instead? Write a new job description for your former inner critic. Find a way to work together, instead of against each other.

My inner critic's name is....

From now on, they are in charge of . . .

This involves . . .

I no longer need them to . . .

The impostor within

Has your inner critic ever tricked you into believing that you're an impostor?

'Impostor syndrome' is a flavour of anxiety, which centres around self-doubt about our competency. Impostor syndrome is the overwhelming, recurring feeling and belief that you do not measure up to your expected or perceived skills and ability. In some ways, it's as if our inner critic is gaslighting us to not believe in our work and our actions. It tells us whatever it can to make us second-guess ourselves. Impostor syndrome can hit us in our jobs (*I can't do this*), our romantic relationships (*I don't deserve this kind of love*) and other responsibilities that we have.

For example, we all know that Superman can fly, right? It's his undeniable USP that he flies in the sky with a red cape and blue leotard in order to get the bad guys. But what if Superman didn't believe he could fly? It's a crippling feeling to know that others are expecting something that you're not sure that you can deliver. And it doesn't matter how many times you have flown before or how far or strongly you flew before, the self-doubt remains.

Since impostor syndrome is built up by negative self-talk, Superman might see himself as a phoney. His self-doubt will tell him that he's not as good as everyone thinks he is; that he doesn't deserve all of the respect he receives; and that his Superman suit is actually the one that deserves all of the credit. He may even self-sabotage by setting far-reaching, impossible goals for himself to prove his worth.

Impostor syndrome is an internal maze that we can struggle to get out of. When we experience it, we often have difficulty recognizing our own competency and skills, leading us to believe the worst of ourselves. According to Dr Valerie Young, expert and TEDx speaker on impostor syndrome, there are five types of impostor syndrome:

The Soloist – *Asking for help shows that I'm not good enough*

The Superhero – *I'm only good if I'm the best at everything*

The Perfectionist – *It wasn't perfect. I could have done so much better*

The Natural Genius – *I'm not good enough since it didn't come naturally to me*

The Expert – *I'm a fraud because I still have so much to learn.*

With impostor syndrome, sometimes the better we do, the more inadequate we can feel. It's incredible to think that Oscar-winning actress Lupita Nyong'o said even winning an Oscar made her impostor syndrome feel worse. Part of the problem is having a low self-esteem tank to begin with, where we don't believe we can bring much to the table. So we overwork ourselves or outperform to receive recognition or success through external outlets, like awards or promotions. But then when we get there, we attribute our success to external factors like luck or nepotism. Our self-esteem tank doesn't allow us to internalize our own hard work and achievements. We focus in on the win in order to justify our right to be there. But once we receive it, we talk ourselves out of believing that it is a validation of our skill and that we have even more to prove. We focus on achieving conditional positive strokes in the shape of awards, promotions and milestones, rather than just believing in ourselves.

I first heard the term impostor syndrome during my training as a therapist. It was my third year in training and I had just started my placement as a trainee therapist, working with children in a primary school with my first-ever therapy clients. Despite having three years of knowledge under my belt, I felt like a complete fraud. What the hell was I even doing here? I found myself meeting with parents and teachers, questioning how much they could see I was undeserving to meet with their children. Whilst they were kind and smiled at me, I imagined that they were scrutinizing my age, my ethnicity and my right to be a therapist. Maybe they thought

I was too young, too dumb or too quiet to be trusted with these children. I was convinced that they were on to me, and soon I'd be pulled out of my placement because of it.

I looked at my peers. And even though some of them were saying the same thing, I didn't believe them. In my mind, I felt they were better than I was. They had more rights to be a therapist than I did. I visualized their confidence in the therapy room and imagined them doing the most beautiful, moving therapy work whilst I felt like a mumbling, fumbling mess of a therapist. That's what impostor syndrome does. The belief that you might have fluffed your way through leads you to doubt yourself and your capabilities. Despite positive feedback that I was receiving, and more importantly the meaningful relationships I was having with my clients, I didn't believe I was good enough.

There are a few key ingredients that make some of us more prone to the anxiety of impostor syndrome than others:

Newness: Whilst it is normal to feel out of your depth at a new job or in an environment which sits outside your comfort zone, this feeling didn't leave me for a long time. In fact, four years later and fully qualified, I still felt it despite having over 500 clinical hours under my belt by that time. And even now, almost 10 years on, I feel it whilst writing this book. What the hell can people learn from me, impostor syndrome says.

People-focused work: It turns out that impostor syndrome is very common for people who work in helping professions, such as therapists, teachers and social workers. That's because their work is unmeasurable for the most part. When there is no script, no ruler or code to follow directly, we struggle to measure ourselves and our performance.

Authoritarian parenting: Having controlling or overprotective families where perfectionism and high-achievement expectations are set, means that these values are written into our inner critic and affect how we view and measure ourselves. Perfectionists set goals that are impossible to reach. If they do reach them, they spoil and undervalue the accomplishment and so are constantly dissatisfied.

Minority groups: Impostor syndrome also most commonly impacts women and people of colour. We only have to Google *impostor syndrome celebs* to see the endless strong, successful, female and/or people of colour who share their experiences of feeling like a fraud in their field. Tina Fey, Maya Angelou and Michelle Obama, to name a few. Comedian Amy Schumer once said she felt like a tourist in Hollywood.

For me, this suggests how impostor syndrome is less about competency and more about our position in society or sense of belonging. Gender, race and age are all determining factors for those who experience the feeling they do not belong in a space that they've worked hard to be in. When we achieve a status and don't see other people who look like us, it leads us to doubt our right to be there.

Being one of the few people of colour and the youngest person on my psychotherapy course, I struggled to find a sense of belonging, leaving me to question my right to be there and my abilities to be a good psychotherapist. I compared myself to my white female peers, who in my eyes could walk the earth much more gracefully than I was allowed to as a young Black woman stepping into the very-white psychotherapy world. When you are the 'only', it adds a pressure to represent for your group.

The truth is, the version of ourselves that people hold in

their minds is none of our business. We don't need to carry the responsibility of other people's expectations of us. Instead, we need to look inward and remind ourselves of who we are and who we are becoming. We need to look at ourselves without judgement and remember that we are capable of incredible things. Because, to paraphrase Mindy Kaling, Why the hell *not* me?

You do you, boo

Building our confidence so that we feel good about ourselves no matter what takes a lot of time and patience. We need to let go of the many years of tying our worth to the wrong things, like our work, beauty or what we offer others. Whilst many people will tell us to fake it until we make it, the best thing that we can do is to start from the bottom up. Giving ourselves the positive unconditional strokes that our younger selves always needed is how we build our confidence as adults.

The more that we centre the needs and expectations of other people, the more we move away from being confident with our authentic selves. We need to have our own back by being our own biggest supporter, so that we give ourselves positive strokes from the inside rather than from the outside. So from here on, I encourage you to be your biggest cheerleader, your loudest spokesperson and your most compassionate caregiver. You will love yourself for it later down the line.

Here is a healing formula for growing our self-esteem and confidence.

Lens Check

Low self-esteem is like wearing shit-tinted glasses, where our vision is so clouded with negativity that we can't see our true reflection. If we've been given a lifetime of negative strokes and course-correctors, we learn to internalize and see that version of ourselves. We absorb the projections that don't actually belong with us. You have had to see yourself through the eyes of other people for so long. You will never meet all of their standards, and actually you never should have to. So let's check and change the lens that you're looking at yourself from.

Start by thinking about all the things that people have told you about how you should be. Write them down and slowly assess each one, asking yourself, *Does this fit who I am and who I want to become?* This will help you to set a barrier between who you are and how other people want you to be.

We can also shift our lens of our work and our creativity. Rather than looking down at our work as something that is not good enough, we can look up to it as inspiration. Asking questions with the view of learning from your work can start this shift. Such as *What did I enjoy or learn from this project?*

Taking a lens check might also involve letting go of comparison. You, my dear, are one of one. You should never have to be anyone but yourself, and comparison will only have you believing otherwise. In the words of RuPaul, 'Impersonating Beyoncé is not your destiny, child.'

Learning how to fall

We spend so much energy trying to be good, right and perfect. These are the three wishes of our ego, which can have us in a chokehold. When we constantly strive to be good, right and perfect, we learn to only equate our self-worth to achievements and success. By allowing ourselves to be messy and make mistakes, we start to let go of achievement as a measurement of our worth. We start to value the meaning of something, instead of the achievement of it. We start to fall in love with the process and how we feel when we do it, instead of what we hope to achieve from it. How our life *feels* is more important than how our life *looks*.

So here is your permission to practise being bad at something. Yes, I said what I said. You could do this by finding a new hobby or activity which you have little knowledge about. You might choose something that you fear or that you imagine you will be bad at. You are not defined by what you are good at, and nor are you defined by what you are bad at either.

As a kid, I was terrified of roller-skating. My fear was about the shame I might feel if I fell whilst roller-skating. My fear was being bad at roller-skating and everyone seeing just how bad I was, so I totally avoided it. Until recently, when I decided that I need to kick that fear in the butt. I decided to take up roller-skating classes and I experienced a sense of fun that I couldn't have expected after my years of fear. And can you believe what the first thing the teachers taught us? How to fall. Learning how to fall taught me how to let go and to step into my joy. Because I knew how to fall safely, I could let go of standards of perfection and hold on to the joy of skating. And guess what? Sometimes falling gives us the opportunity to rise up and see where we stand.

Different Strokes

It's never too late to fill our self-esteem tank with different strokes. We can give ourselves the unconditional positive strokes that we always needed now. Doing this on a regular basis will add unconditional positive regard to the way that we speak to ourselves internally.

We can do this by being intentional. Intentional about what we're listening to, such as finding power songs which fuel our confidence at the start of each day, and the culture we consume. And being intentional about catching self-critical thoughts – ask yourself: would you be comfortable saying the same thing to a friend? To assist in this process we can also tap into the practice of using affirmations. Affirmations are new scripts which hold us with positive regard. They challenge limiting beliefs and reshape the thoughts that we have about ourselves.

Whilst we are filling our self-esteem tank with different strokes, it's important that we scan to see who else has access to our tank. If we've grown up with critical or shaming parents, it's likely that we will also attract critical and shaming friends into our circle. It's important that you have a transparent moment with yourself to look at the people in your orbit. *Who praises you? Who believes in you when you're finding it hard to believe in yourself?* Draw closer to those connections.

Now, who drags or pulls you down? Who shows envy or party poops when your joy shows up? Start to observe those connections more closely. And if you find yourself often feeling not good enough when you meet with those people in your life, it's a sign to talk about it with them or to draw back completely.

It's time to change the way that you speak to yourself and who writes your script.

Exercise: Who's Your Fairy Godmother?

Our inner critic is very much part of the furniture in our internal world. A piece of furniture that we can't dispose of because it comes with the house. However, we can give it less of a focal position in our living space. One way to do this is to give more attention to the other inner parts that we have access to.

We've already met the inner child, the inner parent and the inner critic. But there are many more parts of us. Some are more vocal than others, but they all have the same goal:

to protect us. Though not always successfully, as we know from our inner critic.

Let's give the mic to a part of us that can go head to head with our inner critic. Someone who I call the fairy godmother. As we know from fairy tales, the fairy godmother is a maternal figure with magical powers. She acts as a guide and mentor to the main character, like a godparent might in real life. Fairy godmothers are generous and warm and add a balance to the presence of wicked stepmother. Enlisting an inner fairy godmother can be a great antidote to balancing out the presence of our inner critic.

A gentle note that this might feel awkward or silly at first. But remember that practise makes things stronger. So here are a few questions to get you started:

Name one person (real or fictional) who would be the ideal fairy godmother for you. This needs to be someone who exudes warmth, kindness, wisdom and maybe even humour. Take a mental snapshot of them.

What is it about this person that makes you feel warmth and encouragement? Write down something they say that makes you smile.

What would they say if they were face to face with your inner critic? How would they back and support you? Write a list.

Do this a few more times with other fairy godmothers, godfathers, godparents. The more the better.

When your inner critic is being harsh, come back to this list.

At the heart of every wobble we have with our self-esteem, it's so important to remember who we are and what we're capable of. Because if you really looked at yourself in the mirror without expectations or pressures, you would see the truth: you are *always* enough.

Real Talk on Self-Esteem

- Self-esteem is about how 'good enough' we feel.
- We all have a self-esteem tank that needs filling with good, positive strokes.
- The more positive strokes we received in childhood, the more good enough we feel.
- Our inner critic is the harshest part of our inner voice, and is made up of times we were criticized in the past.
- Impostor syndrome is an internal maze that we can get stuck in.
- We can learn to be more confident and self-loving by shifting the focus and expectations we have on ourselves.

8

Love and Relationships

*Nobody is born with a natural skill of
being able to love themselves.*

Drag icon RuPaul says, *If you can't love yourself, how in the hell are
you gonna love somebody else?* Which is great advocacy for self-
love, but it can make some us feel worse rather than empowered.
No-one is born with a natural skill of being able to love themselves.
It's something we have to continuously learn and work on.

Ideally, we would have started our lessons in healthy love
as kids. Growing up in a loving childhood home or having
encouraging teachers would have gifted this to us. We absorb
these lessons in love and they become the makings of us and how
we love. But what if we've never received safe, consistent love?
How do we access something that we never had to begin with?

For some people, their environment led them to feel unlovable
and so self-love was a myth. This was out of their control and
had nothing to do with their lovability factor. But sometimes
experiencing the genuine and safe love of someone else like a friend,
partner or therapist can give us the tools and vision to love ourselves.
We can internalize that love and give it to ourselves when we need it.

Friendships and romantic relationships have the potential to be our second chance of learning to love and be loved. Having the safety and intimacy that we didn't have as children can help rewire our brain, so that we develop a more secure attachment style. Healthy relationships, romantic or not, have the power to reverse the negative ways that attachment trauma moulds our brain and our behaviour.

The more good love we experience, the more oxytocin our body has rushing through it. A beautiful biochemical of love, oxytocin is a hormone and neurotransmitter which brings us the warm fuzzy feeling that comes with love, sexual desire and mothering. But above all, oxytocin promotes safety, builds trust and *blocks* fear. Yep, I said it. These key ingredients of safety, trust and fear-fighting energy are a recipe for post-traumatic healing, especially the healing of relational trauma. This is why attachment styles can change over time, because we can learn to feel more safety in our relationships with others thanks to more exposure to oxytocin and healthy bonds where we feel validated and loved for just who we are.

Being loved by a partner, even if we didn't feel loved by our parents or previous partners, can transform the way that we see and love ourselves. We're not doomed and two truths can co-exist: we can be hurt in relationships but we can also heal within a relationship. That's not to say our partner needs to mend us, but experiencing safe, reliable love in adulthood can create the right temperature to repair the wounds from the lack of it in childhood.

What's your type?

Do you have a type or is your brain just going with what feels familiar from your childhood?

A common question that clients ask me in therapy is 'Why do I always attract the wrong people?' It's important that we keep our hearts open for new people, but it can be disheartening if new faces continue to open up the same old wounds again. It can feel like feeding ourselves to the wolves.

And if we didn't get all of those needs from our parents, we grow to become especially sensitive to them.

Most of the time, we don't choose the partners we need, we choose the parters who feel familiar. Our brain usually believes that what is familiar is also safe. It's like walking past McDonald's when you're on holiday in a country that you don't know very well. Seeing the familiar golden arches puts a smile on our face and if we're hungry enough, we might step in for something to eat. With relationships, the familiarity can be on such an unconscious level, that we don't really realize until shit hits the fan. We might choose a partner who treats us, loves us or neglects us the way our parents did. That's because we have a set of behaviours that we learned from our parents that then fit like a glove when we meet people who are similar. So if our parents are our unconscious compass for our friendships or romantic partners, of course we will continue to find the same type of people over and over again.

Even where we now have more access to a pool of suitors via online dating, the people that we click on are based on this sense of familiarity. Sometimes when we do meet the right people for us, we might even get the ick. This is because we are being shown someone who is different from what we know. It raises our amygdala alarm system to say no to taking the risk. We have to also remember that when we meet someone who is different from what we know, it's likely that we will also meet parts of ourselves that are different from what we already know. *Maybe this person might actually be a person that will stay? Maybe they will actually love all of me? And maybe they're someone that I could actually learn to trust and depend on.* For many of us, and especially if we've had relational trauma, it can be scary to feel close to our needs being met. There could be more vulnerable parts of us waiting ahead, and that could raise fear or the ick.

Real Talk Moment:
- *What is your type? What are some common themes across the people you are attracted to or have dated in the past?*
- *What are some of your icks? These are things which make you feel instantly unattracted to someone.*
- *What might these say about the relationships your brain is attracted to the most?*
- *Where does that come from?*

Attachment, again

One way of shifting the cycle is by making sense of our own attachment behaviours and how they show up. In chapter 2, we found out about the attachment patterns that we form in childhood which can follow us into adulthood. For a recap, if attachment styles could talk, this is what they'd say:

- **Secure** – I feel comfortable being open and close to my partner. I miss them when they're away but I don't feel worried.
- **Avoidant** – I don't feel comfortable being too close or too open to my partner. I find it hard to depend on them so I'm self-reliant when they're away.
- **Anxious** – I want to stay close to my partner. When they're away, I fear that they'll leave me because they don't love me as much as I love them.

Our parents are our first teachers of what love should look like, and this follows into our friendships and romantic relationships. We unconsciously expect that we need to navigate adult love the way we did in our childhood. This means that in every relationship we walk into, we bring our childhood needs with us. And so does our partner or friend.

Sometimes we meet people who can pour love into the needs

of our attachment. But other times, we meet people whose attachment style triggers our own (and vice versa).

Let's look at some of the ways that anxious attachment behaviours show up within ourselves and our friends or partners.

Avoidant Attachment

When overwhelmed, they respond with withdrawing behaviours like:
Not responding to text messages
Suspicious when things get too emotionally close
Ghosting
Not sharing what they're feeling
An attitude of 'Plenty more fish in the sea'

Anxious Attachment

When fearful, they respond with protesting behaviour like:
Panic or jealousy when there's been distance
Giving a lot and settling a lot
Tries to control when feels threatened
Double-texting
Worries about being abandoned or disappointed

The trickiest relationship of all can be between an avoidant attachment style and an anxious attachment style. Each of their attachment behaviours both triggers and attracts the other.

Let's imagine Fatima and Jamal are in a relationship, and they've just had an argument. As someone with an avoidant attachment, Fatima wants space to decompress after the argument. She doesn't deal with conflict well, as she grew up watching her parents give each other the silent treatment. So she doesn't text or call Jamal the next day as they usually would do. In fact, she turns her phone off for a few days for some quiet. Her hope is to sit alone with her feelings until they subside and she's ready to text Jamal again

Jamal on the other hand is in a panic. After the argument, he's left holding worries about whether Fatima still loves him. The next day comes and she doesn't call him, which makes him feel even more concerned. He checks her social media and sees that she's also gone quiet there too. He wonders who she is spending her time with instead of him. The uncertainty of not knowing what she is thinking and whether she still wants to be together is unbearable. So he texts her, and when she doesn't reply after an hour he sends another text and another and another. For him, each non-response is a confirmation that she doesn't love him any more.

Now, when Fatima does decide to switch her phone on, she sees a stream of text messages asking her for reassurance and to express her feelings. She feels overwhelmed, so she responds back with short and blunt answers, and might even downplay the relationship to escape the intimacy of it.

This type of relationship becomes an Anxious–Avoidant trap. Even when there is a reconciliation, it can often be short-lived before the next cycle starts again. It becomes a bit of a chase, with Jamal needing closeness and reassurance, whilst Fatima needs distance and space.

This doesn't mean that these two attachments can't work together. It just means they need to take more careful consideration in attending to each other's needs and triggers.

What an avoidant partner can do . . .	What an anxious partner can do . . .
• Communicate in a kind way when they need space. Agree a time of when you will reconnect • Practise being more emotionally available to yourself and others • Give yourself permission to have your feet firmly in the relationship • Give your anxious partner reassurance.	• Give yourself space to pour into your own needs • Give yourself permission to have your own hobbies and interests outside the relationship • Reaffirm your own boundaries • Ask for reassurance and transparency about how they feel about you.

There is a saying in the Bible that before you point out the speck in someone else's eye, you need to look at what might be obstructing your own eye first. Before we look at our partner's attachment style as a problem, we first need to look and understand our own. As we've seen with Jamal and Fatima, each partner's own attachment behaviour rubbed the other's the wrong way. So it's important to ask yourself, what is being re-enacted right now that I need to attend to? How do I respond from a place of clarity, rather than from panic or overwhelm?

This is why falling in love can tap so deeply into old childhood wounds. Our families are our first teachers of loving and being loved. If our parents didn't openly show love for us, we won't be able to recognize signs and communications of love from our romantic partner. It can be harder to trust someone who does communicate their love to us and we might find ourselves testing this over and over again. On the other hand, if our parents abandoned or rejected us, whether that's physically or emotionally, then we're going to be left with greater fears that our love interest will do the same too. When this happens, we find ourselves pushing love away before it pushes us away because we grew up to expect nothing more than disappointment and hurt. Or every time they're not in our presence, we go into a panic that they will forget, betray or leave us. Essentially, the way that we were loved becomes the blueprint for how we expect to be loved.

Conflict's not all bad

No matter how hard we try, sooner or later conflict naturally shows up with the people we love. Considering all that we've already said about how complex our personal stories can be, it would be almost impossible for our stories not to collide with someone else's at some point in the relationship.

Some of us grow up to be conflict-phobic: we withdraw or avoid confrontation at all costs in our friendships, romantic relationships, at work, everywhere. This often happens because somewhere down the line we learned that disagreements always end in disaster. We might have seen this with our parents, or with our siblings. It's also possible that our flight trauma response taught us to shut down our needs because speaking up about them brought us trouble and pain. Or our fawn trauma response tells us to gloss over conflict by leaning into people-pleasing instead. But compromising our own needs in a relationship isn't an act of nobility. If we've held on to unsaid things, it adds an additional fear that the verbal diarrhoea of pent-up anger or frustration might take over our mouths. We can run from the risk of saying the wrong thing or getting hurt, but that also means running away from the potential of good love too.

On the flip side, some of us grow up to feel attached to conflict. We find ourselves expecting it or even provoking it in different areas of our lives. Conflict and chaos might feel as familiar as furniture to us, and we might even believe they are a confirmation of love. This can happen if we've grown up to see our parents in tumultuous relationships or if that's all we've known in our own relationships. Our fight trauma response is triggered so we react with aggression instead of reflection. When we feel fired up, it's almost impossible to have a vulnerable and productive conversation because our amygdala alarm system is on. And as we know, no deeper conversations can happen when that alarm is buzzing so loudly. Things might escalate quickly and we might say or do something hurtful. But also when we are attached to conflict in this way, we love the honeymoon period that follows it when things are temporarily smoothed over. We find ourselves in a cycle of pain and passion that feels hard to interrupt.

Because of these, we're often made to feel that whenever there is conflict in a relationship, it's a sign that it's toxic. But what if I said conflict in any relationship isn't necessarily a bad thing? Actually, when we survive after conflict, we can thrive after conflict.

Therapists call this *rupture and repair*, where the relationship breaks but both parties are willing and open enough to work towards mending it together. Doing this has the potential to strengthen and deepen the relationship. It's like the Japanese art of *kintsugi*. Broken pottery is put back together again using gold lacquer. Not only does it look stunning, but it shows how we might be able to not only repair the cracks but their resilience might even be the best part.

Another great but revealing thing about conflict in a relationship is that it sheds the layers of projection that we put on our partner. When our partner makes a mistake, we quickly realize that they're actually not as perfect as we projected them to be. They are a real-life human just like us, with their own personal story and their own ripples of healing to get through. Conflict reminds us of this, and that if we want to heal and grow as a couple, we need to speak to each other more deeply. We can't expect our loved ones to be psychic about our needs, we have to communicate them. And let's remember that our needs can change, so an ongoing dialogue has to be at the heart of the relationship.

> *Real Talk Moment:*
> - *What did conflict look like in your childhood home?*
> - *How did your parents deal with conflict between each other?*
> - *If you had any siblings, how did your parents step into your conflicts?*
> - *How do you feel about conflict now?*
> - *What is your response to conflict in your friendships and relationships?*

When conflict is bad

So why do so many arguments turn out so badly?

A relationship without good enough communication is like driving a car without using your indicators: you're destined to crash. Whether it's a friendship or a relationship, conflict will always happen somewhere and it's important that we learn the wrong and right ways to talk it out.

The way that we speak to our loved ones matters.

In the 1980s, relationship psychologist and researcher Dr John Gottman found four key behaviours that contributed to the downfall of our relationships. He called these the Four Horsemen of the Apocalypse.

The Four Horsemen
Criticism
We deal with conflict by verbally attacking their personality through criticism. We use 'You' statements to communicate. e.g. 'I thought *I* was your best friend, but *all you do is* spend time with your boyfriend these days!'
Contempt
We attack their sense of self and assume that we know better than them. Contempt releases any built-up thoughts we've had about them. e.g. 'Don't you think you're being a bit *needy*? It's childish'
Defensiveness
We see ourselves as the victim and project all the blame onto them. e.g. '*I've never* done that to you. *I'm always* available whenever you need me. *You're the one* that won't spend time with me.'
Stonewalling
We deal with conflict by tuning out, withdrawing, giving them the silent treatment or disregarding them. e.g. 'Just forget it. Do whatever you want. I *don't care.*'

So choose wisely. Do you need to be right or do you need a healthy relationship? We might want to be right, but what we need for the relationship to progress and deepen is for both of us to feel heard and listened to. And the door of defensiveness doesn't take us there.

Good, healthy love isn't conflict-free. When we confront our feelings and our needs, we give our relationship an opportunity to grow and blossom. Closed mouths don't get fed, so it's important that we create a culture in our relationship of giving non-judgemental feedback.

Giving (and receiving) feedback

If you are someone that finds it difficult to give honest, open feedback to your loved ones, that's OK. It's never too late to learn and experiment with it, and being in a safe and secure relationship is the best soil to try in. Try the following:

Try writing

If we're not used to healthy conflict, it's likely that our words will get stuck in our throat or they might just come out as venom. If either of these are your fear, the power of writing might be your saviour. Before approaching the conversation, write a list of what issues you are holding on to and what needs are not being met. It can also be helpful to write a list of what things you enjoy, love or feel gratitude for in your partner or friend. By doing this, you're creating some clarity for yourself before you have the conversation by reflecting on what exactly you want to communicate.

And if speaking these out still doesn't feel possible, you might want to try writing a letter instead. Remember that having a healthy relationship is the goal, so make sure your words are kind and curious.

Check in about their capacity

Before rushing in to share your needs and feedback, ask your loved one whether they have capacity. This allows them to have some autonomy in engaging in the conversation, rather than feeling blindsided. You can do this by saying 'I think it would be a great idea for us to talk through what's working and what needs some work in our relationship. When's the best time for you?' Avoid saying 'We need to talk'. Thanks to romcoms and sitcoms, we've learned to expect this means a break-up is on its way. Saying this might cause panic in your partner, leading them to step into the conversation defensively.

The 'right' time

There is never a perfect time, but it is important to find a good-enough time. Avoid giving them feedback when they've just woken up or whilst they're having an already stressful day. At the same time, try not to procrastinate by waiting for the perfect moment to arise. No matter when you do it, it is going to feel awkward and clumsy at first. So forgive the awkwardness and press forward with it.

Walk and talk

If sitting across from each other feels too confrontational, invite your partner for a walk and talk. Walking whilst speaking openly about any issues can dilute the tension for both of you. Nature is good for the soul and can provide a calming atmosphere, with enough distractions if we need to slow down the conversation at any point. Also being in a public space might make you feel more at ease if things do get heated.

Giving options

If your partner comes to you with an issue about the relationship or if they're coming to you for support, it's a good idea to know how to be there for them. Often when our partners come to us for support, we support in the ways that *we* would like to be supported rather than what *they* would need. They might want a cuddle to soothe them following their work stresses, but instead we might respond by giving them practical advice that they never asked for. So when your partner tells you about their troubles you can respond by saying 'I hear you, it's been really tough. Would you like me to give you comfort or advice?' Not only are you giving your partner an option, but you're also creating clarity for yourself on how you can be a good partner in that moment.

Learning how to argue

Instead of using more toxic ways to argue, we can try non-violent communication, a communication model created by Marshall Rosenberg. Violent communication is when we use our words to harm people, like the Four Horsemen approach to conflict. Alternatively, we can try using safe and open language to express our needs and feelings, so that we are moving the conversation towards where we want to go rather than being struck in a triggered and defensive place. We use first-person 'I' statements, rather than blaming or projective language. There are four steps.

1. Observation: In a non-judgemental way, state the facts of what you noticed. Avoid blame and words like 'never' or 'always', as they overgeneralize and assume your side of the story is the right side. Doing this without making any assumptions will prevent the conversation starting from a defensive place.
Instead of: 'You never spend time with me any more.'
Try: 'I noticed we haven't had any quality time together this week.'

2. Feelings: We can take ownership of our feelings by naming them. It's important to remember that another person's actions cannot *make you* feel anything. Their actions might prompt what you feel, but it's our current needs and past baggage that cause us to feel as we do. We can open up by sharing our feelings or asking our partner about theirs.
Instead of: 'You made me upset. You're so selfish.'

Try: 'I felt anxious because . . .'
Or: 'Are you withdrawing because you've been feeling stressed at work?'

3. Needs: Connecting our feelings with our unmet needs helps to move us towards improving the relationship. Return to chapter 1 for the list of needs.
Instead of: 'I want you to be home more.'
Try: 'I need quality time together so that we can build our relationship.'

4. Requests: Suggest a request or solution. This request needs to be clear and conscious of what you are asking for. It should also be focused on something that you want, not something that you don't want.
Instead of: 'Stop spending so much time at work.'
Try: 'Could we have an hour together in the evenings when we're both home from work?'

This structure can be used in most contexts, whether it's asking your partner to do the dishes more often, setting boundaries with a friend or giving feedback to a colleague. And if things do get heated, agree on a safe word to communicate when things have gone too far.

For things to work in a relationship, both parts needs to be doing the work. It's impossible for one person to carry the relationship alone on their back. When this happens, they're eventually going to buckle and fall, forgetting themselves and their needs in the process. We can do all the backflips and cartwheels we can to try to maintain the relationship. But if our partner isn't meeting us with a similar effort, we do ourselves and our self-love a disservice by staying. Just because someone can't love you the way that you need doesn't mean that you're unlovable. Their capacity doesn't match yours and that shouldn't mean that you need to make your needs smaller. But it does mean that you may need to let go of something that will never really fulfil your romantic appetite. Sometimes love in a relationship isn't enough. In order to have self-love, we sometimes have to break our own hearts by leaving a relationship that doesn't meet us where we are.

Heartbreak

Sometimes good things actually need to fall apart so that better things can come together. Love isn't always enough to hold a relationship together, and we have to make the choice to say goodbye to someone we love. Romantic and friendship break-ups can be among the most painful things we can experience. And if you haven't had a broken heart before, there are millions of songs that teach us just how painful they can be.

The power of deciding the fate of a relationship can put us in a state of agonizing ambivalence: 'Should I stay or should I go?' It can feel like an impossible choice to make. Choosing to stay in a dead relationship can break our heart just as much as choosing to leave one. So many relationships eventually go kaput after weeks, months or years of dragging out the finality of announcing the end. Sometimes we've emotionally left the relationship a long time before we've even said the words. Our emotions walk away before we have the words to verbalize them.

Being the first person to initiate a break-up can be a guilt-provoking experience. The worry about inflicting pain on our spouse can leave us feeling like the villain. And in many ways, we might be seen as one. Regardless of the circumstances, we exist in a society where the person who called off the relationship receives the wrath of the community that exists around the couple. Friends and families project onto them as the villain, whilst the receiving spouse can often be seen as the victim in the situation. In reality, it takes two people to have a relationship and both have their own part to play in the accountability of its demise.

Initiating the end of relationship is also terrifying because, well, what if we get it wrong? Even in a toxic or unfulfilling relationship, we might worry that we are saying goodbye to the best relationship that we will ever have. We might even begin to gaslight ourselves by invalidating our doubts about the red flags in the relationship, and decide to power through. But the safety of staying in a dead relationship takes us away from the potential of finding a live and healthy one. If we choose to stay in a relationship to avoid abandoning a partner, we will end up abandoning ourselves in the process.

The end of a relationship, and I would say especially the end of a toxic one, can be one of the most emotionally painful experiences we have in life. It throws us into grief, except the person we're grieving is still fully alive and accessible with the click of a button. We can even stalk their social media if we miss their face or want to see what their life looks like without us. It's savage. How do you grieve someone who you still have physical or digital access to? The longing and loneliness can lead us to spiral back into the arms of an ex, sidetracking our process of grieving the relationship.

In fact, a break-up can activate the same parts of the brain linked to addiction and also reduces chemicals in our brain and body like dopamine and oxytocin which usually make us feel good. This leads us to have withdrawal symptoms from our ex, like low mood, tremors, vivid dreams and inability to sleep. We can feel a similar pain and craving when separating from a partner as we might from substance withdrawal. And relapsing by returning to a bad relationship might give us the dopamine dose that we've been craving, even if it eventually turns sour again.

The end of a relationship also triggers a very young experience that we've all had before: separation anxiety. Most of us grew up with at least one primary caregiver who we grew close to or dependent on to meet our needs. As we explored in chapter 2, we would have been enmeshed with them for most of our early years. But there would have been a time where we were old enough to go to childcare. Quite suddenly, we found ourselves removed from the familiarity of our secure base and the person who made us feel safe to a very different environment with new sounds, sights, people and other kids. This can be a shock for children who struggle to make sense of whether mummy or daddy has abandoned them in this strange place. And even when their caregiver does come back, they might cling to them in fear of losing them again. This separation anxiety is normal for kids, and we see it for most of the children in the strange situation experiment I explained earlier (see page 30). So as an adult with a broken heart, our feelings might unconsciously time-travel right back to that moment of being left behind in a strange and scary place. We regress back to needing them close to us, even if they caused us pain. It becomes a cognitive dissonance that the very person that we want to be comforted by is the same person who we feel hurt by. So don't forget to give love to a part of you that feels scared and won't let go.

Messy break ups

Ten years after their break-up, Monica couldn't understand why she wasn't yet over her ex. The end of their relationship came like a ton of bricks when they were in their mid-twenties. Monica had not expected it at all, and they had a messy few years of casual sex and unmet promises to reconcile. Until one day when her ex announced that he was seeing someone else.

Monica felt betrayed and rejected, but, wanting not to be 'difficult', she agreed that they could remain friends. To be honest, this felt like their only option. They had known each other for so long that they shared the same friendship group even ten years later. Messy as this was, understandably Monica couldn't part ways with these friendships. Leaving them behind would have left her without a support network to grieve her ex, even if he was also a part of it. In therapy, we unpacked how being in the same friendship group made it feel like nothing had changed. It was like sharing a bedroom with her ex where all the furniture was still in place. Every time she spent time with her friends, ex included, it tricked her brain to believe that nothing had changed and they were back together. And so every meet-up broke her heart all over again. It also meant that she had no space or permission to let herself be separate from her ex. Sharing the same friends restrained her from exploring her own sex and dating life away from her ex, in fear of what information would filter back to him from their shared pals. We worked together to think about what boundaries and distancing she needed to put in place from her ex and from their shared community.

Monica's break-up shows just how complicated the end of a relationship can be. No relationship is just two people. Saying goodbye to a partner might also mean saying goodbye to a home, a community, safety and resources. And this is even more complicated if we have children, animals or other dependants within the relationship.

Friendship break-ups can be just as hard, if not harder than romantic ones. Our friends are the people who know us the most intimately, and usually from a much younger age than our partners do. Most of the time when this does happen, it's because the friendship has somehow turned sour. So it can feel confusing or like a betrayal when a long-time friendship eventually breaks down. And the person to whom we would normally turn for comfort is no longer available. Time changes people, and it's normal to outgrow our friends, but it doesn't make it any easier. So yes, friends can break our heart too.

The person that brings us comfort is the very same person we need to grieve. Even in a toxic relationship, the dopamine hit of being reunited and back in the honeymoon phase is tempting for a broken and grieving heart. The reality is that you can't heal by going back to the person who broke you.

Advice for healing a broken heart

- I trust that the end of your relationship was for the right reasons, and so the first thing I'd like you to know is . . . Congratulations on your break-up! Honestly, this is something that we do not do enough. But you deserve the credit and kudos for making or being part of such a hard but necessary decision. Allow yourself to pay gratitude to listening to yourself. Find the good in goodbye.

- Remember that two truths can exist at the same time. You can love someone who is also terribly wrong for you. You can hold anger for someone, whilst also holding love and longing at the same. Even when our heart has been shattered by them, we can still love someone with all the tiny pieces that we have left. Heartbreak is complicated and we can feel many, sometimes conflicting, things all at once. What we feel and what we need might be at war with each other at times. Allow both to exist so that you can reflect and process them.

- Sometimes we have to create our own closure. When we haven't been given context or reason from the person that we loved, it can be really confusing and leave us with questions that might not ever get answered. Create your own closure by reflecting on what you think were the final chapters of the relationship. Do this without projecting blame on your ex and without putting all of the accountability on yourself either. Focus on non-judgemental observations to come up with a conclusion of where the story ended.

- Grief work is a big part of dealing with a break-up. Treat this almost like a death and allow yourself to go through the motions of different feelings like sadness and denial. Remember you will not only be grieving the person you were in a relationship with, but also that particular part of your life and what it represented for you.

- Even though that relationship is over, there are parts of you connected to that relationship that should continue to exist. Whether it's reclaiming songs that you shared with your ex, or particular hobbies, they don't just have to belong to that relationship. Those things can have new memories and new meaning, so reclaim them as your own.

- Only start dating when you feel absolutely ready and have the right reasons. Dating because you feel lonely or bored or envious of friends in relationships is not a good enough reason. In fact, these reasons might lead you to attract the wrong suitors in your life, because you're seeking someone from a place of needing to fill or compensate for something. Continue to do inner work on yourself. And when you feel you have clarity and space in your heart for the best love of your life, go for it.

- Can we ever get back with an ex? So many of us have experienced that feeling of still being connected with an ex, something that is often called a soul tie. Depending on the context and the individuals, reconnecting with an ex can either be a blessing or a disaster. What makes or breaks a reconnection with an ex is how much inner work both people in the couple have done since the initial break-up. Enough self-work from both people has the potential to mend the relationship that once was, like the gold lacquer of *kintsugi*.

Exercise: Date Yourself

Whether we are single, dating or in a relationship, it's important that we keep expressing love to ourselves by giving ourselves our own time and words of affirmation. This practice of 'dating ourselves' is important in helping us to love ourselves before we expect anyone else to do it for us.

So here is your gentle reminder to take yourself out on a date. It could be a nice meal, a day at a coffee shop or even a fun activity you've been wanting to try.

Dating is also about getting to know someone deeper and showing our appreciation. So here are some creative prompts to help you do that:

List five things that you love about yourself that are not based on your appearance.

What qualities in yourself do you enjoy the most?

What are your dreams?

What would the past version of you think of you now?

Name something about you that you keep falling in love with.

(P.S. This is great to use before going on a date with someone, especially if you feel nervous.)

Where's the stretch?

Healthy relationships need to stretch in order to grow. In their book *Big Friendship*, Aminatou Sow and Ann Friedman describe stretching as the way that friendships adapt to new circumstances. For example, a small stretch is having a friend who's a new parent, which means they're not going to respond to your messages as promptly as they used to. And a bigger stretch is having to renegotiate the terms of that friendship entirely because their new parenthood means their priorities have had to change.

Life throws a lot of curve balls at us. You are not the same person as you were yesterday, and you're yet to meet the person you will be tomorrow. It only makes sense that as we're growing and healing as individual humans, our social connections need to come along on the journey. The more stretch there is in a relationship, the more space there is to welcome the person we're becoming.

This happens a lot when we're healing. Through unpacking our stuff and getting to know where we've journeyed from, we might realize the ways our false self was showing up instead of our true selves. We start to see the ways we were being the person that other people needed us to be, and leaving ourselves out in the process.

When we start to heal and grow closer to becoming more like our real selves, it can create a rupture in our social circles. This might happen if:

- You're not as 'fun' or sociable as you used to be
- Maybe your priorities or interests have changed
- You're standing up for yourself more
- You're more emotionally available and wanting to talk about deeper emotional things
- You've made lifestyle changes
- You've let go of toxic patterns and toxic roles.

It's possible that you don't seem as 'fun' as you used to be in their eyes. It's natural for this to be a surprise to the people who have known the past versions of ourselves. It's likely that you'll both need to grieve the person you used to be.

But a healthy friendship will have permission to stretch in embracing the new, Real Talk version of you. Not limiting you to staying as a version of you that suits them. Sadly everyone you love won't be able to grow with you.

So ask yourself, what is the stretch like in your current friendships and relationships? Where do you feel there is enough stretch to welcome your healing? Where do you feel like there is no stretch and the relationship is about to snap?

How much we give out

As much as stretch *within a relationship* is good, overstretching ourselves without reciprocity isn't. While our community and our relationships are important to our wellness, we also need to take some responsibility in how much we pour into them. By this, I mean we need to stop expecting people to give us what we're not willing to give ourselves.

Because when we're able to give ourselves the love that we deserve, we stop loving other people from a place of survival and past trauma. And if there's one thing that we can all benefit from, it's boundaries . . .

Real Talk on Love and Relationships

- Healthy relationships, romantic or not, have the power to reverse the negative ways that attachment trauma moulds our brain and our behaviour.
- Our brain is attracted to people and relationships who feel familiar from our childhood. Our brain is also repelled by people and relationships that feel too new and unfamiliar, even when they could be fulfilling.
- The trickiest relationship of all can be between an avoidant and an anxious.
- Conflict is necessary in relationships and doesn't have to be toxic.
- The way we speak to our loved ones matters.
- Criticism, contempt, defensiveness and stonewalling are bound to break a relationship. Using non-violent communication is bound to strengthen a relationship.
- Heartbreaks, including friendship heartbreaks, can be some of the toughest things we'll experience, but we can always heal through them.

9

Boundaries

We can't nourish someone else,
if we're malnourished ourselves.

I sn't it funny that one of the first words we ever learn as toddlers is the same word that so many of us struggle to say as adults? The word 'No'.

It can be a trying moment for our parents – especially saying no to everything offered to us – but a powerful moment for us. It's the first time that we realize we are separate beings from our parents, with separate thoughts, feelings and needs. So we – very enthusiastically – say no in order to exercise our newfound autonomy and individuality. Because it feels good to make our own decisions about what we want and what we don't want. Playing with boundaries as toddlers helps us develop our sense of true self.

But somewhere along the way, we lose this sense of freedom and it becomes a lot harder for us to say no to things. We might feel guilt, pressure or a fear of disappointing others, leading us to silence our 'No'. We can end up compromising the sense of freedom and free will that we previously had in order to keep others happy. We lose hold of our boundaries.

Let's talk about boundaries

Boundaries are the expectations and guidelines that we set for ourselves and our relationships. Boundaries are the line that shows the limits and capacity of our relationships. We use boundaries to teach others how to treat us and how we should treat them. They help our relationships feel good.

Imagine that you have a bubble around you. This bubble represents your personal space, needs and capacity. What sits within our bubble is everything that makes us feel safe, comfortable and secure. It's the secure base that we create for ourselves. Having a firm and safe bubble around us gives us a strong sense of our needs and choices. We feel strong because we know exactly who we are by having a healthy boundary in place.

When you look around, you realize that everyone else has a bubble around them too. Their bubbles also make them feel safe and comfortable. And when you interact with them, your bubbles meet. This meeting point is the boundary that we need in a healthy relationship. Boundaries help us show love to others whilst also loving ourselves. How do we love somebody else without losing ourselves in the process? Boundaries are about bringing us close enough together while retaining our personal space. When we have healthy boundaries with others, we can equally communicate our needs and strengthen the relationship between our two bubbles.

Our bubbles and the bubbles of other people equally deserve to exist and be respected. We can take care of our bubble, whilst also being respectful of other people's bubbles. They don't need to change their bubble and we don't need to change ours. Our bubbles don't need to merge either. Even though it would make us feel closer to each other, it wouldn't make either of us feel safe or comfortable and there wouldn't be enough space for us to be our own person either.

And even if we think someone's bubble looks exactly like our bubble, it isn't. Our needs and capacities are so individual, requiring us to each have our own individual set of boundaries. We don't all see the world the same way. What is comfortable for one person and their boundaries can sit uncomfortably outside another person's boundaries. For this reason, we can't assume what somebody else's boundaries are, or that somebody knows our boundaries, without us clearly telling them.

There are lots of different types of boundaries that we need in different areas of our life to preserve our wellbeing and mental health. These include:

Physical boundaries: how we set rules around our personal space, our home and physical touch. For example, being mindful about who you do and don't feel comfortable having in your room.

Relationship boundaries: how we allow ourselves to be treated and what behaviours we accept from others. For example, choosing to not be friends with your ex-partner whilst healing from the break-up.

Emotional boundaries: how we allow others to make us feel, how much of other people's emotions we take on and our emotional capacity. For example, noticing which friends only contact you when they want emotional support, but are not willing when you need it.

Time boundaries: how much time we give to others compared to how much time we give to ourselves. For example, work eating into time spent on ourselves.

Material boundaries: how we set limits around the relationship we have with money and how we lend or borrow money or possessions with others. For example, excessively rigid or reckless spending habits are a sign of messy financial boundaries.

Sexual boundaries: how we communicate what does and doesn't feel good with sexual intimacy and what we feel comfortable and ready for. For example, ensuring that you feel physically and emotionally ready before being sexually intimate with someone new.

Moral boundaries: how we respect and practise our morals, values and spiritual beliefs. For example, being a feminist and dating someone who is openly misogynistic would compromise our moral boundaries.

Most of our boundaries are context-dependent and flexible by nature. As we grow and heal, we move towards knowing ourselves better. Our needs change all of the time and so do our boundaries. However, we can also have deal-breakers, boundaries which are non-negotiable for us. These types of boundaries are for things that would uncomfortably press against or burst our own bubble. If we accept a trespass on our boundaries, it's almost as though we've lost a sense of self because it goes against our core values. These compromises to your hard boundaries could include deciding whether to forgive a partner after infidelity, having a friend that uses racist language or tolerating abusive behaviour towards you. They can put us in a whirlpool of confusion because whilst we love this person with all our heart, accepting their behaviour may no longer make us feel safe and secure in our bubble. And what we accept from other people is also a reflection of what we accept within ourselves.

> **Real Talk Moment:**
> - *Make a list of some of your non-negotiables. These are things that would clearly cross the line for you.*
> - *Think about what non-negotiables you have in relation to friendships, work, dating and your body.*

What moulds our boundaries

Our first teacher of boundaries is the bubble of the womb we were created in. The womb gives us warmth and nourishment, in tender walls. The boundaries of the womb fulfilled all of our needs while also allowing us to grow and be born. And even though we are inside the body of our parent, we're not totally consumed by them.

We are still our own person, while our mother is also her own person. So even from the beginning, the boundaries of the womb taught us that we were our own person.

Too many of us then grow up learning to compromise our boundaries. As kids, we might have been told to kiss and hug relatives we hardly knew even if we didn't want to. We are rewarded when we are 'good girls' and 'good boys' who follow the rules set out for us. And when we decide to question or rebel, we are 'bad girls' or 'bad boys' who are shamed and punished for having a mind of our own. Society tells us it's good to be compliant.

There are a number of reasons why we might have a difficult time with boundaries. These include:

Unhealthy boundaries in childhood
If we grew up with inappropriate boundaries, we may have inappropriate boundaries as adults. Children learn from what their parents do. Having parents who don't provide healthy boundaries leads us to not know how to give ourselves healthy boundaries. Whether we had overly strict, authoritarian parents or lenient, enmeshed parents, it can lead us to build spiky or wobbly boundaries. It can often happen that we develop the opposite of what we received, e.g. someone who grew up with rigid boundaries may end up with wobbly boundaries in search of the flexibility they always wanted, but on the extreme end.

It's important to remember that how our parents set boundaries for themselves also teaches us what to do with our own boundaries. E.g. how did our parents protect their own self care?

Trauma
As we know, when we've been through trauma, our body gets activated into survival mode. Our Inner Batman doesn't want to be vulnerable ever again, which can lead us to build some spiky boundaries. On the flip side, trauma also impacts how

we understand ourselves and view the world. We might be less connected to our bodies, and therefore less able to know where our capacity and our boundaries lie.

Societal pressures

Society encourages us to compromise our boundaries all the time. One of the ways that it does this is through hustle culture, where we are constantly encouraged to prioritize productivity and entrepreneurial success over our mental wellness and right to rest. For example, if we work in a toxic work environment where it is normalized to work late hours and never take annual leave, we will feel more pressured to choose to do the same.

Neurodiversity

Boundaries can be extra complicated for those who are neurodivergent, and there's a few reasons why this is the case. First it can be difficult for some neurodivergents to know what they need since they may have some trouble processing their emotions. Some people with ADHD, for example, can have a tricky time due to absorbing other people's feelings quite easily. This double empathy can make it hard for them to untangle outside feelings from their own. Some neurodivergents might also find it confusing navigating the nuances of different people's boundaries, which could cause more anxiety in social relationships. Lastly, many people under the neurodiversity umbrella had to spend a lot of their lives masking in order to fit neurotypical expectations. This means there is another layer of compromising their needs in order to fit with the mould of wider society.

As a therapist, boundaries have become the heart of my own self-love and healing. Helping people through their personal stories and trauma can be fulfilling work, but it can also be emotionally draining when I'm pushed to my capacity. It means that I need to be protective of my emotional rest and social time outside of being in the therapy room with my clients. I discovered this the hard way through my social life. As I started to tell people that I was training to be a therapist, I found myself attracting more and more people wanting to trauma-dump on me at social events. (Trauma-dumping means oversharing difficult information without the other person's consent or during inappropriate times without considering how your words impact the listener.) As soon as I shared my job title with someone new, I would somehow be caught up in a conversation about their childhood trauma or broken relationships without my consent or invitation. As an introvert, I can find most social events depleting, but this was a new level. These connections felt one-sided and emotionally draining for me, and I would end up emotionally burned out in the days that followed. Each time, I also felt myself boiling up with resentment because people were assuming my boundary as a therapist meant I had an endless capacity to talk to people about their trauma at a casual houseparty on a Friday night. My needs as a person were not being considered. So from then on, I stopped disclosing my job to new people. By setting that boundary with myself, I built in time to get to know them and share more about my job gradually whilst working out their understanding and consideration of personal boundaries.

My boundary is that I only keep friends in my life who allow emotional reciprocity. I have great girlfriends who feel like sisters where we can always be there for each other. Some of them are therapists and some of them aren't. But with each of them, there is a mutual understanding that I can lean on them and they can lean on me. However, we always check in first by saying something like 'Hey, I'm having a bad day, do you have capacity to talk?' Not only does it give me a heads-up, but it also gives me the autonomy to check in with my own capacity before being honest about whether I can support it at that moment or not. Saying no isn't about rejecting that person's feelings or that bad day. But it is about being honest with them and ourselves. We can't nourish someone else if we're malnourished ourselves.

My boundaries will be different from your boundaries and your boundaries will be different from my boundaries. And that's OK. We are too beautiful and unique to be fulfilled and nurtured by the same emotional guidelines.

How boundaried are your boundaries?

We might have even experienced trauma where elders disrespected, disregarded or invalidated our boundaries as children altogether. When these things happen, we learn to toughen or weaken our boundaries. The shape of our boundaries might end up being what I call spiky or wobbly.

Spiky boundaries are when we don't allow any flexibility or nuance to our boundaries. Instead they can be rigid and can also keep other people at arm's length in order to protect ourselves. Spiky boundaries lead to . . .

- Not sharing our personal story
- Seeing everything as a red flag
- Being a closed book
- Feeling overly comfortable with silence or allowing other people to take up all of the space
- Not giving others a chance to understand our needs
- Giving little of ourselves in relationships
- Difficulty saying yes to others
- A tendency to 'stay out of other people's business'
- Making decisions based on rigid principles
- Cancel culture or cutting someone out of our lives when they make a mistake, no matter how small.

On the other side of things, wobbly boundaries are when our

boundaries are too flexible, because we move them or they are easily breached. We end up being enmeshed with other people and not having a clear understanding of our own selves. Wobbly boundaries lead to . . .

- Oversharing our personal story
- Ignoring red flags
- Being an open book and sometimes trauma-dumping
- Difficulty with silence and saying more than we wanted in order to fill it
- Being dependent on satisfying others' needs before our own
- Giving all of ourselves to others
- Difficulty saying no to others
- A tendency to take on other people's problems as our own
- Making decisions based on what other people are doing
- Always going with the flow
- Never having a consequence when people breach our boundaries and making excuses for their behaviour.

Both spiky and wobbly boundaries aren't good for us, since neither of them support us in communicating our needs or maintaining a strong sense of self. It's also possible that we might have spiky boundaries in some parts of our lives and wobbly boundaries in other areas. For example, we might have spiky boundaries around dating, where we are discerning with our romantic interests. But at the same time we could have quite wobbly boundaries around sex, impacting who and how we get our sexual needs met.

Real Talk Moment:
- *What type of boundaries did you have in your childhood home? Were they spiky, wobbly or healthy?*
- *What boundaries did you grow up to have yourself?*
- *How do you think that happened?*

People-pleasing

Nobody finds boundaries harder than the people-pleaser. People-pleasing is a behaviour where we prioritize being nice, polite and kind over being truthful with ourselves. This might not sound too bad, but in reality people-pleasing is the false self at its finest. The problem is that being nice, polite and kind are traits which are deemed admirable in society, as they should be. But for someone with people-pleasing tendencies, they end up doing this at the expense of themselves. When we don't trust ourselves or don't take our needs seriously enough, we end up putting the needs of other people first. When we people-please, we allow ourselves to move our boundaries for other people.

People-pleasing isn't based on love, it's based on fear. It is often born out of the fawn trauma response, which we mentioned in chapter 7. This is a survival technique from our brain which helps us diffuse danger in the atmosphere by appeasing the needs of others, playing on humour and being likeable so that we're less likely to be harmed. We learn the fawn response from being in unsafe environments or unsafe relationships, protecting ourselves by being nice and conforming. If we're fearful of an attack of criticism or rejection, we do all that we can to rectify it through changing ourselves for the other person by matching their energy, for example. But falling into fawn for too long creates our tendency to people-please. We need to eventually learn that we're safe now to be in our own skin.

The thing is that it can also be a form of self-sabotage. By taking the responsibility to please someone else to maintain a safe connection, we are actually losing our authentic selves. For example, many of us put on our best selves when we're dating someone new, but this is especially the case if we have people-pleasing tendencies. We try to match up to what our romantic interest desires, sometimes playing a part. But it doesn't matter how much we shape ourselves to fit their type, it will eventually be noticed that something is missing. And that something is our authentic self. We may end up feeling resentful towards our romantic partner because we can't express our needs or they might feel resentful at us for suddenly having needs.

The tendency to people-please shows up as . . .

- Difficulty saying no
- Over-apologizing
- Fear of what people will think of you if you ask for help
- Fear of disappointing others
- Hiding your authenticity in order to be liked (self-censorship)
- Responding to calls and text messages instantly
- Over-explaining yourself when you make a mistake
- Excessive guilt when you practise self-care
- Feeling that people take advantage of your time or kindness
- Believing people can't function without your input
- Giving more than your capacity
- Settling for less than you deserve
- Taking on someone else's truth
- Excessively using humour, vulnerability or kindness to connect with people
- Over-committing to things (e.g. agreeing to take on a new work project when you're already at capacity)
- Talking yourself out of your real thoughts and feelings
- Depending on praise to feel valuable
- Feeling like a burden
- Feeling responsible for other people's feelings or their experience
- Steering clear of making decisions
- Saying yes and then feeling resentment later
- Sharing too much of yourself to make other people feel comfortable.

Does the nature of people-pleasing feel familiar from some of what we've talked about before? It showed up when we learned about the guilt wound of our inner child. It also showed up in some of the dysfunctional family roles, like the family clown who has to make everyone laugh to help their family escape emotional conflict.

Life as a people-pleaser can feel like a duck gliding on water. From the outside, they're smiling and coolly gliding with ease. But under the surface, they're kicking their feet like hell to meet the expectations of other people, while also masking all of the effort. A people-pleaser hardly ever asks for help because they are fearful that this will make them less likeable and less needed. And so they never want to make a fuss.

Until I started therapy, I had no idea about my own people-pleasing tendencies. My secret goal was to be my therapist's favourite-ever client. For a long time, I found myself only saying what I thought my therapist wanted to hear. I came to therapy looking pretty and polished with a full face of make-up, silently praying for a compliment. I tried to impress her by cracking jokes and with all of my psychobabble and (ironically) my self-awareness. And when she asked me about difficult feelings it made me feel uncomfortable because I didn't want my feelings to make her feel uncomfortable, prioritizing her experience over my own. This is what happens with people-pleasing. We focus on what other people need of us while ignoring what we need of ourselves. I was thinking about her bubble, instead of thinking about mine.

Eventually, in her own kind way, my therapist told me to cut the crap. We unpacked how my need to be her favourite tied back to Little Me, who was scared of being forgotten. But I was forgetting myself in the process. So I began to (reluctantly) challenge myself to being less polished, making more space to invite the messy, no make-up, serious and sad versions of me to sit on the couch. Because the truth is I wasn't in therapy for my therapist, I was there for me. The same way you are not here reading this book or living life for anyone but you.

As Brené Brown says, boundaries are about taking the risk to love ourselves whilst potentially disappointing others. But disappointing others is often the deepest fear for someone with people-pleasing tendencies. And so we end up giving those people unlimited access to ourselves. Other reasons why people-pleasing can make boundaries difficult include:

- Fear of conflict
- Fear that others will be angry at us
- Fear of being seen as difficult, mean or selfish
- Fear of ruining the relationship
- Fear of authority
- Assumptions about how we think they will respond
- Believing we can show people how to treat us instead of telling them.

As a result, we often move our boundaries for other people, especially if we think they are older, wiser and more influential than we trust ourselves to be. In the shadow of a giant, we might expect that disappointing someone else is more disastrous than disappointing ourselves.

If you are someone who is prone to people-pleasing behaviour, I want you to know that you do not need to set yourself on fire to keep everyone around you warm. It's not necessary to sacrifice yourself in order to care for others.

Reclaiming your boundaries as a people-pleaser can feel like tipping out your backpack and realizing that you were carrying heavy items that never belonged to you in the first place. We can notice how much other people's stuff has accumulated over time, getting in the way of our own. Instead of choosing burden and obligation, you can step into your autonomy and liberation.

We are worth more than just the crumbs left over from our own love and care.

Exercise: A People-pleaser's Brainstorm

Learning how to reclaim our no is the most powerful thing that we can do as our healing from people-pleasing. Because if we don't protect our own capacity, who will?

Often it can be a natural first instinct to say yes to a request, rather than giving ourselves time and space to assess our actual capacity and whether we want to add this request to our responsibilities. We might find it hard to say no on the spot. Instead, we can try slowing down our people-pleasing tendency by using what I call a Please Pauser. Please Pausers help us to delay our response so that we can have time to think about our answer instead of answering on the spot. For example, by saying 'Let me come back to you on that', we create a delay so that we can go away and think about our boundaries before communicating it at a later time.

Brainstorm some Please Pausers of your own, some ideas would be:

Let me come back to you on that

I need to check my schedule first

We underestimate our capacity by not asking ourselves the right question first. Here are some of the questions that you need to ask yourself before agreeing to take on a commitment. For example:

Do I have space in my life for this?

Do I want to have space in my life for this?

How much joy, safety or fulfilment will it bring me?

Learning the power of our 'no'

Nobody can set boundaries for you except you. We can't expect other people to tell us where our limit should be and we can't expect them to guess either.

Setting boundaries can be difficult and uncomfortable work. But it is also one of the most rewarding and fruitful things that we can do ourselves.

One thing that stops so many of us setting boundaries is that we're worried it will come across as rude. But boundaries don't need to be mean or rude. In fact, they're an act of love and kindness as we're showing someone how to respectfully love us. By choosing to say no to some things, people will know you really mean it when you do say yes to other things.

Once we become more comfortable with the language of boundaries, its power ripples through to the other parts of our lives. It becomes a skill that we carry with us in the rest of our healing. While life will always have its ups and downs, the one thing we can always have control over is communicating our boundaries. Here are three healthy habits for nurturing boundaries:

#1 Listen when anger shows up

Anger is a boundary's best friend. It's what we feel when someone does us wrong. We feel it when we believe we are being taken advantage of. So naturally, anger is one of the first things we'll feel when someone has crossed, disrespected or ignored any of our boundaries. Anger is our body's way of standing up for ourselves. Our boundary is being crossed and the feeling of anger steps in to fight for us.

We've been told that anger is a bad emotion that needs to be managed. But there is often truth to our anger. It won't be the undoing of us, but it will be the undoing of our people-pleasing parts.

Resentment is another emotion to look out for, a cocktail of anger and regret. We often feel resentment once we've given too much of ourselves to someone and saved very little for ourselves. When we feel resentment, it's usually a sign that we broke our boundary for the needs of somebody else. Sometimes we do this because we wanted to be praised for it or we expected them to do the same for us. But that's not how boundaries work.

Be with anger and resentment before sending them away. You might want to take pen to paper to express and see them in front of you. Be curious about where those emotions are coming from. What boundary was broken? Or what boundary did we break for somebody else? Does this remind you of a broken boundary from your past?

#2 Choose you

We may have experienced a lifetime of pushing our own needs to the back of the queue, and so it feels like second nature.

When we invalidate our own needs by making them seem less important than they are, we are in fact gaslighting ourselves. We do this by making excuses for other people's behaviour, ignoring our intuition, believing we are asking for too much or minimizing our feelings.

But you are not being dramatic, or oversensitive, or too much. You are simply figuring out how you want and expect to be treated going forward. It may feel completely foreign and vulnerable to say *Yes, I deserved better and I always have.* But your intuition said what it said, so take the time to listen to it and the boundaries it's urging you to reclaim.

#3 Say it with your chest

Now this is the part that you've probably been dreading. Sooner or later, you're going to have to give your boundary a voice. We can't dance around it or leave hints for others to guess our needs. The only way to set a boundary is to say it. No, we need to bite the bullet and say it with our chest.

It wouldn't be fair for us to expect someone to know or guess what our boundaries are, even when it feels obvious to us. We all have a different, distinctive set of boundaries. What is a hard no for you might be a hard yes for me.

For example, a physical boundary for me is that guests have to take their shoes off at the front door when they visit my flat. This is something I picked up from my family home and from the homes of all my relatives, so I grew up assuming this was everyone's boundary. But visiting other homes as an adult taught me that my boundary was probably a cultural one. So at first, when friends from different cultural backgrounds to my own would walk straight into my home with their trainers or boots on, I stayed silent and angry. On the one hand, I knew it didn't sit right for me. But on the other hand, wasn't it a bit ridiculous to ask them to take off their shoes? Was it a weird thing to ask someone if they didn't grow up with the same house rules? What if they didn't feel comfortable? Would they think I was insulting the cleanliness of their shoes? I didn't want to make them feel uncomfortable in my home.

Eventually I realized that entering my home should also mean respecting the boundaries of my home. Leaving shoes at the door is a house rule for me that keeps my home a home, and a respected one at that. So the next time those friends came over, I said, 'So good to see you. You can leave your shoes in the hallway. Let me know if you need any socks.' And it was totally fine, and no one ever needed to question it.

This simple boundary fulfils what I believe are four things we need to be when setting boundaries. These are:

Be kind: 'So good to see you . . .'
Boundaries are an act of love and can be spoken about in a kind and loving way. It's always best to teach someone our boundaries in a non-defensive way. You may want to start by sharing words of appreciation to the person or to the actual relationship.

Where possible, avoid setting a boundary whilst you're in the heat of anger. In fact, set a boundary with *yourself* to not set a boundary whilst in the heat of anger. Impulsively saying things without considering them could lead to both of you feeling more hurt than needed.

Be clear: 'You can leave your shoes . . .'
Sometimes when we're communicating our boundaries for the first time, we end up sugar-coating them so much that the person isn't able to see what it is we're asking. We do this because we're fearful that they'll think we're being mean or that they'll be mean to us. It's our fawn response kicking in to soften the imaginary blow and gloss over any conflict we're expecting. It can also be incredibly vulnerable to put our needs out there in the open, especially if our needs have been rejected in the past. But by beating around the bush, our boundary can get lost in translation.

If we want someone to take our needs seriously, we also have to take them seriously by communicating our boundaries in a clear and serious way. Boundaries are about saying what you mean. Remember, say it with your chest, without having to hide or sugar-coat.

Be specific: 'in the hallway . . .'
Being specific might feel pedantic and extra, especially if you're not used to clarifying your expectations in a relationship. But because we are all so different, we can each have different interpretations of the same boundary. For example, you might set a boundary with

a friend, asking them to stop calling you so late at night. But what is 'late at night' for you might be interpreted differently for them. We can't assume that everybody sees the world exactly the same way that we do. In this case, being general isn't helpful for us and it definitely isn't helpful for them either. So don't be shy to say your specific limit, e.g. no calls after 9 p.m.

Being clear and specific is like providing instructions for a recipe you want them to complete. The more precise you are with your boundaries, the easier it will be for your person to know how to respect them.

Be supportive: 'Let me know if you need any socks'
Remember when we spoke about rupture and repair? By showing support at the end of communicating our boundary, we are bridging the gap between us. We are saying *I'm telling you how you can love me and my bubble because I still want to be connected with you and your bubble.* It is a nudge of reassurance that the relationship is OK despite a boundary being put in place.

These nudges could look like offering them resources or alternatives to help them respect your boundary, an invitation to talk about what happened or offering to reconnect at a later time if either of you need space.

Obviously, most of the work that people need to do around boundaries is a lot more complex than asking someone to take off their shoes indoors. But the same strategy can be applied to most boundaries. Here are a few examples:

An old friend has started to make sarcastic remarks that don't make you feel good:

'*I care about our friendship a lot. But that comment you just made doesn't feel good to receive. And it's not the first time. When you say those things, I feel a friction between us. Can we talk through it?*'

A family member keeps asking when you will get married or have children, leaving you to feel pressurized:

'I know you want the best for me, but I don't feel comfortable having this conversation.'

You're dating someone new and they suggest taking things to the 'next level', but you don't feel ready yet:

'I love where this is going, it feels good getting to know you more and more. I'm not quite ready to take it to that level just yet though. I like you, but I also need more time for our connection to keep growing. What are your thoughts?'

Boundaries can also sound like . . .

- I can talk for twenty minutes
- Thank you for asking, but I'm not available
- I respect your opinion, but this is my decision to make
- I can help, but not in the way that you're asking
- I understand that you're upset, but I do not want to be spoken to in that way
- Right now, I really need some space. Let's talk about this tomorrow
- I'm not able to help this time
- I'll respond on Monday
- If this continues, I won't be spending as much time here.

Apart from our two-year-old selves, no one is great at setting boundaries for the first time. It will feel clumsy and awkward and messy at first. It's also likely that guilt will show its face, telling us not to take care of our own needs. But guilt doesn't mean you should resurrect your wobbly boundaries. Remember, practice makes it stronger. Keep nurturing the root need and your capacity to set boundaries will grow. Allow yourself to experiment with your boundaries language in different arenas of your life.

Let me be real with you by saying not everyone is going to like your boundaries. Most people will be taken aback, surprised and even defensive, especially if they're not used to hearing you be honest about what you need. But after some time to digest, I hope they will take the necessary steps to meeting the needs of your bubble.

And how about when someone crosses the line or refuses to honour our boundaries? It's not uncommon to lose relationships after setting a boundary with them. This can be sad, painful and frustrating. However, if anything, it is a sign of how much that boundary needed to be in place. You deserve people in your orbit who honour and validate your needs. And anyone who was unable to respect your bubble does not deserve to take up your space being connected with it.

It is not because you asked for too much, but more likely that they are not enough for you. As long as you were kind, clear, specific and supportive, you did absolutely nothing wrong. Perhaps when you addressed your needs it highlighted that they had some unaddressed needs of their own . . .

Whilst it might hurt to say goodbye to those relationships, it is their loss. It's better to lose a relationship than to lose yourself.

I once heard Gabrielle Union say in an interview that there is no better anti-ageing beauty secret than water and setting boundaries. They preserve our energy and help us live the life we deserve.

No matter what we go through in life, boundaries are a choice that we can make to navigate the drama in our lives. As a client once told me, we get to choose to jump off someone else's merry-go-round.

Exercise: Boundary Check

In the following image, map out how healthy you feel your boundaries (see page 182) are. Wobbly boundaries are at the centre, spiky boundaries are at the edge and healthy boundaries in the middle. Where would you plot your boundaries with your work, friends, romantic relationships, finances/material possessions?

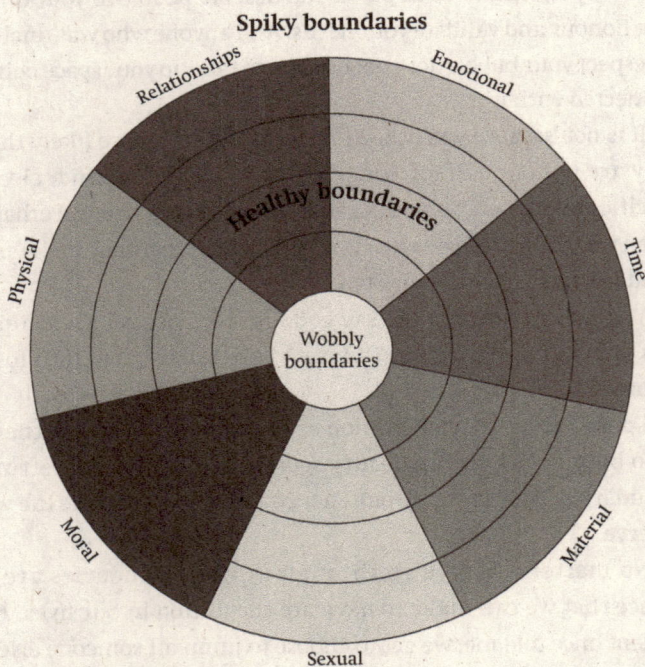

Spiky boundaries

Relationships

Emotional

Healthy boundaries

Physical

Time

Wobbly boundaries

Moral

Material

Sexual

What boundaries do you need with others?
What boundaries do you need with yourself?

Real Talk on Boundaries

- Boundaries are the limits we set that helps us feel safe and our relationships feel good.
- There are different types of boundaries, including non-negotiables which are things that would clearly cross a boundary for us.
- If we don't have healthy boundaries, they might be spiky (inflexible) or wobbly (too flexible).
- People-pleasing leads us to move our boundaries for other people.
- A starting point is learning how to pause before we say yes to things we would probably want to say no to.
- Anger and resentment let us know when we need a boundary in place.
- To set boundaries we need to be kind, clear, specific and supportive.

10

Body Image

Our relationship with our body is the
longest relationship we will ever have.

Y et it's also the part of ourselves that we judge the most.
Take a moment to think about the relationship that you
have with your own body. How do you speak to your body? What
conversations do you have? What are your best moments with your
body? And what are your worst?

One reason why we give our bodies such a hard time is that our
body is the first thing anyone notices about us. Naturally, we all
do judge a book by its cover, which means we also judge people by
their bodies. Nobody wants to admit that, but it's our brain's way
of figuring out someone new. We look at how they're dressed and
how they carry themselves. But we also unconsciously look at their
physical form: their complexion, hair colour, their body shape. It's
our primitive brain's way of figuring out *are you like me?* Because
when someone looks like us we feel more at ease and familiar. We
have found someone that we belong with and so we can take a sigh
of relief. But when we come across someone who doesn't look like
us, this can unconsciously make us feel a spectrum of threat. We

zoom in on the details that separate us. And often, we compare and contrast ourselves using what society sets as our measurement of comparison. So it becomes a competition of who fits society's rules best. Desirability politics has us competing against each other for attention, attraction and respect, often defined by the male gaze.

When we feel we don't fit the quota for society's expectation on beauty, we internalize the message that we are not good enough. We tell ourselves stories about how 'not good enough' our bodies are, time and time again. *I'm too big. I'm too small. I'm too short. I'm too tall. I'm not beautiful.* We tell these stories to our reflection in the mirror, engraining the narrative over and over again. And the only thing our reflections can do is look back at us and agree.

This is especially the case if we already have a tough time with our self-esteem, like we talked about in chapter 7. The harsher our inner critic and the more rigid our perfectionism, the tougher we are on our bodies. So many of us have an idealized version of our bodies in our minds which we compare and contrast to ourselves over and over again. Over time, we keep perfecting this internal image of ourselves, which means that it would always be unattainable even if we tried. It's the reason we hear of people who change their appearance but still feel dissatisfied and unconfident.

The thing is, the stories that we tell ourselves about our bodies don't start with us. So in this chapter, we will look at how diet culture and body shame get in the way of us seeing just how good enough our bodies actually are. Your body was never the problem.

How we learned to shame our bodies

Can you believe that we had to *learn* to unlike our bodies? None of us stepped out of the womb believing that we didn't look good enough.

We learn it through conditioning, through what Carl Rogers calls *conditions of worth*. These conditions of worth are the rules and expectations that we believe make us worthy and lovable, and can apply to how much love we think our body deserves. A person's conditions of worth might say *I have to be slim to be attractive* or *I have to be smaller or bigger than my partner to be lovable.* Obviously, we were not born with these rules and expectations. But we would have been conditioned by them the moment that we entered the world.

When we carry strict rules and expectations about our body, we end up carrying the burden of body shame. Body shame is the belief that *my body is bad.* When we feel body shame, we feel unhappy with the body that we have and we believe changing our body will make us happier. We try to shrink our insecurities by shrinking ourselves, physically or emotionally. We use the mastery of distraction in order to blend in with everyone else.

There are at least four places where we learn these body judgements: diet culture, social media, family life and our personal experiences.

Diet culture

The world does a good job of telling us what we should and shouldn't do with our bodies. I often tell my clients that 'should' is the language of shame. What we are told about how our bodies should be shames us for how they currently are. Our teachers on this front are the media and people around us who tell us how we should eat, move, dress and have sex. Our bodies aren't acknowledged with grace or compassion, but with rules and boxes.

This is thanks to diet culture. Speaking with author and body-confidence influencer Alex Light, she describes diet culture and fat phobia as 'the persuasive and insidious belief that thinness is more important than physical, mental and general wellbeing and fatness is an objectively bad thing to be avoided at all costs'. And this belief system has been around for hundreds of years. Even the ancient Greeks would restrict their food to gain a sense of self-control and calmness, and since then, dieting is a consequence of fat phobia and body-shaming. Films like *Bridget Jones's Diary* told us that someone who is a UK size 12 would not be happy until they lost weight. Research shows how 71 per cent of plus-sized women are fat-shamed on regular dating apps. And while diet culture tells us what our bodies should look like, it earns billions of dollars from our insecurities even today.

Diet culture tells us the thinner we are, the happier we will be. But what actually happens is we end up feeling not good enough and blame our bodies for how we feel, instead of the culture surrounding us. We might have also internalized some toxic messages too, such as:

- Some foods are 'good' and some foods are 'bad'
- We need a 'summer body'
- We need to be thin to look good
- We should quantify our food (into calories, number of meals day, dress sizes, how much protein/sugar/etc.)
- We should exercise at least as much as we eat
- Our bodies need to be changed or controlled to fit societal ideals
- Thin is good, fat is bad
- We can 'treat' ourselves, but we can't over-indulge
- Healthy means being slim.

Studies show how even girls as young as six years old already have a desire to have slimmer bodies. The messages of diet culture are so subtle that we absorb them from a very young age without even knowing. After recovering from an eating disorder, Alex recalls seeing 'the famous Kate Moss line "Nothing tastes as good as skinny feels"' which 'negatively shaped my belief system around my own body'.

Our happiness has nothing to do with the shape of our bodies. But it will make us unhappy trying to fit to what society wants, especially if we have to harm our bodies to get there. With diet culture, we are never good enough or valuable enough. Diet culture tells us that there's always more we could do to look better and be more lovable. This is the opposite of self-love, where we love ourselves just as we are and the only change we need is change that will bring us healing.

Detangling health from thinness helped Alex to decide for herself what healthy looks like. Alex kindly urges us to turn to compassion when it comes to unravelling our relationship with diet culture. 'Take it easy and treat yourself with the compassion you'd give to someone else. For most of us, this is lifelong conditioning and it's incredibly difficult to unpick. It's OK to be stuck in diet culture, it's so normal. But it's also OK, when you're ready, to slowly start to challenge what you believe about your body.' She also suggests following people of different shapes and sizes on social media, to see a whole range of people embracing their bodies. She says, 'I began to see the beauty in those bodies and that ultimately opened the way for me to see the beauty in myself.'

Real Talk Moment:
- *What messages do you carry from diet culture?*
- *When you were younger, what celebrities did you look up to?*
- *How did they influence your own body image?*

Social media
As awesome as social media can be, it can also be a nightmare for body confidence.

You can't go on social media without coming across perfectly curated pictures, showing someone's perfectly curated life and appearance. And this can be so disheartening to see, especially on days when we were already feeling our worst. As much as we want to feel happy for our friends or the celebrities and influencers we follow, we're likely to end up comparing the appearance of their lives with the appearance of our own. Especially when it comes to how we look.

Remember what I said earlier about the idealized version of ourselves that exists in our mind? We keep perfecting this image over time, and social platforms make it even easier for us to do this. So much of social-media content is so cleverly filtered, and it looks so realistic that we wouldn't know it's false. Filters can now change our face shape, eye colour and even parts of our body. So we end up comparing ourselves and building our idealized image based on flawless pictures of people, when they don't even look like that themselves. And these images ignore the messy, imperfect reality.

With social media, we have more eyes on us and some people can have pretty horrible things to say. It is too easy to be at the receiving end of trolling and cyberbullying, where people leave hurtful judgements and comments about our body on our social media. It also puts more pressure on us to be picture perfect, to protect ourselves from being criticized if we're not.

I know it can be hard to be surrounded by images telling you how you and your body should be. But I want to remind you that another person's beauty is not an absence of your own. And just because a person's picture looks perfect, it really does not mean that their life or their relationship with themselves is perfect. We don't get to see the reality or the mess behind the picture because it gets edited out. If there's anyone that you want to aspire to be, let it be the most healed and self-loving version of yourself.

Family life
Because of decades of diet culture and the objectification of female bodies, there are generations of women with poor body image and insecurities. This means that for many of us, those messages made their way into our family homes. This can show up as intergenerational family cycles of difficult relationships with body image, food and fat phobia.

How our parents treat their bodies has a ripple effect on how we treat our bodies. So if we didn't have parents who unconditionally loved their body, we will be less likely to unconditionally love ours. It's likely that neither did *their* parents, and all their ancestors before that. In my experience of working with clients with disordered eating or a fear of fatness, they almost always have a parental figure who has a tough time with their own body image.

It's an intergenerational pattern that gets repeated until it's generationally repaired. Children see and learn from what their parents do. Having a parent who puts high value on their appearance and the need to diet or change their body makes us develop a lens of seeing our own bodies as something that needs to be changed. The same goes for unhealthy eating habits and toxic relationships with food. Our first teachers of consumption are our caregivers.

Let's imagine being a five-year-old child watching their mother getting ready in the mirror. First, let's imagine our mother smiling and complimenting her own reflection, paying affirming respect to her own body. What would that feel like for a five-year-old child and how would they learn to speak about their own body when they look in the mirror? Now, imagine being a child watching their mother frowning and scrutinizing her own reflection in the mirror. She tries to flatten her stomach or hide her arms because she doesn't think they are good enough. What would *that* feel like for a five-year-old child? And what messages would they pick up about how to speak to their own bodies?

Alex Light agrees that 'it's incredibly difficult to build confidence and self-love on a foundation of self-loathing and feelings of inadequacy when we fall short of that very narrow beauty standard, hence why there are multiple generations of women in particular who are very lacking in self-esteem and self-confidence'. But when we give kindness and grace to our bodies, we can break generational cycles of body shame.

Exercise: Patterns of Body Image

Take a moment to think about your family members and
things they've said or done that give you some clues about
the relationship they have with their bodies. Think about:
Things I know about my siblings/cousins and their
relationship with their body.
Things I know about my parents and their relationship with
their body.
Things I know about my aunts/uncles and their relationship
with their body.
Things I know about my grandparents and their relationship
with their body.

What similarities or differences are there across the
generations?

Our personal experiences
Sometimes we are directly told that our bodies are not OK. If this
happens in childhood it can be a devastating blow to our self-
esteem and confidence in our bodies. Every time we hear directly
or indirectly how our bodies should be, we are told what parts
of our bodies can or can't exist according to other people. Often
comments about our bodies are projections from other people
trying to mask their own body insecurities. Their body shame or
anxiety is projected onto us.

The problem is we often look at our body in pieces, instead as
a whole. We focus on the individual parts of our bodies without
respecting the whole picture. How many times have you looked at
a specific body part, putting it under the microscope to be viewed

by your inner critic? Maybe it was your stomach, your arms or the way your chin looks when you laugh.

These experiences lead us to do what I call 'zooming in'. We start to micro-manage our own bodies, comparing them to the perfect ideal we have in our minds. Since criticism and control are shame's ugly stepsisters, we start to look at our body with the negative view that we need to control and change it.

My earliest body-shame memory came from my years of learning ballet as a child where I always received the same feedback. *Tuck your bottom in, Tasha.* Every single time. And boy, I tried. I squeezed those glutes so tight every ballet class, but would still hear the same five words. *Tuck your bottom in, Tasha.* I looked around and noticed nobody else received that feedback, just me. The expectations of what a ballerina should look like were being projected on my body as a child just wanting to have fun in ballet class. It deflated me and I wished I could make myself, especially my bum, smaller to avoid being criticized for it every week. I couldn't shrink externally, so I started to shrink internally by becoming quiet in class or positioning myself in the corner of the room each week.

With my adult eyes, I now know that I was the only one to receive that feedback because I was one of the few Black girls in that class. Because of my ancestry, my body was different from everyone else's and I was made to feel like it didn't belong in ballet. I found myself tensing my bum muscles outside of class, and this is a habit I even had to learn to undo as an adult. I have since spoken to other Black women who also had similar experiences of ballet when they were little. We had to learn to tuck ourselves in to appear palatable to the gaze of the very white world of ballet.

Another body-shame moment that a lot of people might relate to comes through my love of tracksuits and baggy clothing as a teenager. At the age of thirteen, my teenage and rounded body was quickly developing. And as a result, male strangers, young and old, would take notice and make it known. They stared or whistled or tried to speak to me, even when I was travelling home in my school uniform. Even though I was a child still innocent of sex and attraction, I somehow felt like an object of desires that weren't appropriate. I still remember feeling uncomfortable and wanting nothing more than to hide my body. I learned that my body was too visible and too noticeable, and to avoid this uncomfortable feeling I needed to hide it. So, just like ballet classes, I started to 'tuck in' my womanly bits by enveloping them in baggy, baby-blue tracksuits and gender non-conforming clothing. The idea of wearing anything that was fitted or feminine filled me up with dread and shame. This is what being objectified does. It casts the shadow of shame and we lose our worth and power by the gaze of somebody else.

Your body is yours and it belongs to you only. And so nobody has the right to comment or project onto a body that doesn't even belong to them. And though it was never our fault that we received that shame, it is down to us to unpack the shame that was sent our way so that we can make space for compassion and kindness.

It's time for you to own your body again.

You may notice that you criticize your body most when life feels difficult.

This happened for my client Arlo. Through years of working together, we noticed the pattern that he criticized and punished his body the most at the same time each year: the weeks surrounding the anniversary of the death of his childhood best friend. As a kid, he didn't know what to do with his grief when his friend died, so he began to obsess over the imperfections of his body and coped by over-exercising. And whilst he didn't remember this consciously, his body remembered his trauma. So when those difficult feelings of grief came up every year, so did his poor body image.

Sometimes we confuse feeling bad with our body actually *being* bad. Research shows us that there's a connection between things like childhood trauma or grief and having poor body image or disordered eating. And there's a reason why.

Our body has the brave job of processing all of our biggest and most uncomfortable feelings, especially when we've been through some hard crap in our lives. And let's be honest, these feelings don't feel good. So over time, and especially as kids, we can learn to blame our body for those not-so-good feelings instead of the life experiences that caused them. We internalize the bad things that happened, leading us to see our body as the bad thing instead. We see our body as the problem.

Have you ever come across the phrase 'eating my feelings'? We somehow tangle our emotional needs with our eating habits or the way we see our bodies. We might believe that we're 'feeling fat' or 'feeling ugly', but fat or ugly aren't really feeling words, are they? Instead, we might be feeling sad, lonely, rejected or scared. We use our judgements of our body to tell us how we feel, rather than working in harmony to discover what's happening emotionally under the surface.

Exercise: Letting Go of Projections

When someone makes a projection about our body, it's like they're attaching a label to our body. One label might feel OK, but over the years we might find that our body is covered in labels placed there by other people and without our permission. When we're covered in labels from other people, it makes it harder for us to feel like our body is truly ours. Because we can't see beyond the projections that other people have put on it for their own benefit. Think about: What labels have people been putting onto your body?

How did it feel to receive those labels?

Are there any that you can let go of today?

Are there any that might need more time and healing?

Reclaiming our bodies

Body shame is a sign that we've lost ownership of our body. Someone else's needs, values or opinion has gotten in the way of the relationship. We have to remind ourselves that healing and self-love is about respecting and enjoying our bodies, not changing them.

But it's never too late to fall in love with our bodies again. The good news is there are lots of ways that we can work towards having a more healing and loving relationship with our bodies.

Diversifying our influences

Sadly, culture doesn't show us diverse bodies. We don't get to see a diverse representation of curvy bodies, fat bodies, disabled bodies, Black bodies, Brown bodies, trans bodies and gender non-conforming bodies. When we don't see different bodies that all represent health, wealth and confidence, we learn that not all bodies deserve acceptance.

A great thing about social media is that things are slowly changing. Influencers and content creators are using their platforms to show that all bodies are normal and beautiful and worthy of love. An important starting point for loving our bodies is opening up our eyes to a diverse range of bodies through who we choose to follow on social media, the celebrities that we admire and the books that we read. Embracing the beauty of all types of bodies can help you embrace more tenderness for your own.

Bringing joy to our bodies

An act of self-love is finding enjoyment within our bodies again. We did this as babies, at the very start of our relationship with our body. As curious babies, we used to chew on our toes and play with our body rolls with glee and wonder. We enjoyed the nakedness and softness of our bodies. When we are babies and children, we are totally in love with the bodies we were given. That love was rooted in play, curiosity and acceptance. This is the kind of body confidence that we need to find again.

Coming home to our bodies in this way means that we need to stop zooming in on the details, and start zooming out to see our body's capacity for joy. Joy is the feeling that we have when we align with our true selves. When we finally come home to ourselves, without control or criticism. Joy stops shame in its tracks and tells it to go back to the underworld that it came from. Instead of keeping us small, joy invites us to exist loudly.

We can find joy by giving our bodies the gift to take up space and be celebrated for it. Something that has helped me a lot is reconnecting with my love of dance. I wanted to join a dance class, but I didn't want my body to be shamed like it had been when I was younger. So I joined a body-affirming dance class, designed for and run by plus-size people. And boy, I will never forget that feeling from my very first class. To stand with other people of different curves and shapes, and to see myself amongst such a diverse group, was a sense of belonging for my body that it had missed out on my whole life. Seeing my body move in the reflection on the mirrored wall made me feel so proud and joyful of my body.

I spoke with Trina Nicole, a body-confidence advocate and my dance teacher, who created the curve-affirming dance classes out of her own frustration of feeling unwelcome, ostracized and judged for her own curvy body at other dance classes. Trina says, 'Once you find that space the support and encouragement from your peers really help to alleviate self-judgement and internal ridicule.' These safe, affirming spaces give permission for healing to happen. 'People are always so surprised with themselves. Often, they've never seen themselves like that or been able to express themselves in that way without judgement, so that alone can make people feel vulnerable and bring some emotions to the surface. Dance moves you and can literally help you shift tendencies towards more positive thoughts about your body and improve your overall body image.'

Finding ways to be in a non-judgemental and affirming relationship with your body will open up doors for you to feel joy and body ownership. Dance might be one way for you to explore, but if not, experiment with other ways to be with your body. Maybe it's dance or a way to love on your body, but as Trina says, 'Rediscovering what my body can do is something that I found really helpful. It focused on joyful movement and allowed me to acknowledge that I am strong, capable and my body is pretty awesome.'

Another way to love on our body is to speak to it with the love and kindness it deserves. Your body was born to be your greatest companion, so imagine talking with the same compassion and love that you would give to a friend. This takes a lot of time, practice and leaning into the cringe like we talked about in chapter 6.

Here are some words of compassion and acceptance that you can say to your body on days when it feels tough to hold on to that self-love:

> You are enough
> I feel beautiful
> My body is a vessel for joy
> My body can change but my worth doesn't
> I am so much more than just a body

> *My body is whole and complete*
> *It's OK to take up space*
> *You don't need to be . . .*
> *You're a miracle*
> *All bodies are worthy/sexy/beautiful*
> *I love . . . about my body because . . .*

Also practise giving yourself compliments that are not based on your appearance. Compliment yourself on your wit or creativity or kindness. This can be a nice thing to do with friends too. They might find body image just as challenging as you do.

Protecting our bodies

We also need to set boundaries around our body to keep it safe and respected. This includes setting boundaries with other people who might make comments or offer unsolicited advice about our bodies. Because the truth is, why should anyone have a say about our body when it doesn't even belong to them? Some boundaries we can set when people make comments about our bodies include:

- I don't feel comfortable with having this conversation
- There is more to speak about than just my body
- I don't like when you do that
- My body is not your concern
- What I do with my body is up to me
- It's not my place to talk about your body/not your place to talk about my body.
- My body is the least interesting thing about me.
- My body is not all of *me*.

Exercise: Body Art

Falling in love with our body again requires us to take the time to get to know it again. We can do this by touch, taking the time to explore the many corners and grooves of our form. But one of my favourite exercises is to ask my clients to draw their bodies.

Now this isn't about being good at drawing. We don't need to be artists for an excuse to take in our bodies through drawing them. This is about the process of really viewing our bodies, with appreciation instead of criticism. By drawing or sketching our body, we take the time to view and appreciate it through the softness of sketching and shading.

You'll need to start by taking a photograph of your body. You can take a photo of your whole body. Or you might start with a part of the body that you'd like to learn more about, like your back, legs or shoulders. You may need to ask for someone to help you with this, or to set a timer whilst having your phone held by a tripod or stack of books. Take a range of photos, posed and unposed, so that you have a selection to choose from. Once you've selected an image that catches your attention, it's time to draw.

Create an atmosphere that feels soft and grounding. Music and candles can create a nice setting. Make sure that you have all your physical needs met too, like having blankets and tea alongside you. You can choose any art materials that you feel comfortable with – pencil, biro,pen, paints, crayons or collage.

Spend time drawing what you see of yourself in the photo. Be slow and gentle as you recreate your body on paper, taking in every line, dip and crease of your body. Take as much time as you need but allow yourself to give your full attention to your body.

Once you're done, give your image a title. You might want to give thanks to your body or write down something new that you found out about your body through this exercise.

As Glennon Doyle says, we need to remember that our body isn't supposed to be our masterpiece. It is not our one life-defining piece of work. We are more than just our bodies. Our real masterpiece is finding joy, the whole life that we create for ourselves and healing ourselves to live our best life. What we pour into ourselves and the world around it. *That* is our masterpiece. And the appearance of our body, how thin or fat or curvy or athletic it may be, has nothing to do with that.

Our body changes and our body grows, whether we want it to or not. It will sag when it wants to. It will jiggle when it wants to. It will even slow down when it needs to. The reality of loving our body is realizing that we cannot have full control over what our body does. Our bodies are always going to do their own thing, and we need to respect that.

And Real Talk, life is so much more enjoyable and fulfilling when we focus on doing what makes our body *feel* good, not what we think will make our body *look* good.

Real Talk on Body Image

- We had to *learn* to unlike our bodies.
- When we carry strict rules and expectations about our body, we end up carrying the burden of body shame. Body shame is the belief that *my body is bad* and so we carry strict rules about how our body should be.
- Diet culture falsely tells us the thinner we are, the happier we will be.
- Social media can lead us to have unrealistic perfectionistic standards for ourselves, thanks to filters and editing.
- Body shame can be intergenerational: how our parents treat their bodies has a ripple effect on how we treat our bodies.
- Body shame can be projected onto us, when people mask their own body insecurities by giving them to us.
- We can heal body shame by reclaiming and coming home to our bodies through doing things like centring our joy and diversifying the people we aspire to emulate.

11

Sex

Sex is not a bad word.

Unless we're intentionally going to a sex therapist, sex is often the thing we avoid talking about in therapy. We're more comfortable talking about the murky corners of our past than we are talking about the sexual corners of our bedroom. Even when we've built a safe relationship with our therapist where we can feel comfortable to talk about anything, our sex life is often the part of us that we leave out of our therapy sessions.

I remember when I first brought up sex to my therapist. I felt like a giggly teenager, whispering it as though sex was a naughty swear word. Growing up in a religious household, I had to unpack the ways that I had grown up believing my natural curiosity about sex was sinful or inappropriate. But breaking this down in therapy helped me to let go of judgements I had about sex and build a more sex-positive relationship with myself. 'Sex' is not a bad word.

So what silences us when it comes to openly talking about sex? Our old friend Shame. Shame has been connected to sex in so many ways. We might feel judged for our virginity. Or we might feel judged for not waiting to be married before we have sex.

Or most commonly, we might be judged for our 'body count' and the amount of people we have or haven't slept with. Our sex lives are policed so much by society's tendency to shame. Our ideas of sex have been tampered with by moral, medical and social rules that get in the way of sex positivity. We can be judged for being too sexual or not sexual enough: we're damned if we do and definitely damned if we don't.

Our relationship with sex is just as important as the other relationships in our life. We all have an equal right to the freedom of sex and sexual pleasure. It's one way that we can deepen the relationship with our bodies as well as with our true selves. Physical touch has always been our first language as babies, and sex is one of the ways we speak that language as adults. It can bring us closer to ourselves and the people we feel sexually attracted to.

When it comes to self-love and healing, we can't leave sex out of the conversation. Unlearning the expectations we've built up about how sex should be is just as important to our healing process. And our sensuality is a part of our true self that needs air to breathe and be. Sex has the capacity to bring us more intimately to ourselves, when done within a healthy and healing capacity.

Let's be real, it's not that easy. There are so many things that can get in the way of us having fulfilling sex lives. Most of the time it's how our minds feel about sex. So let's unpack that . . .

Safe sex

So what is the key ingredient for enjoyable sex? Safety. As exciting as sex can be, the starting ingredient always needs to be safety. Whether it's with a lifelong partner or a one-night stand, we need to feel some element of safety with whoever we decide to be intimate with.

Sex and relationships psychotherapist Esther Perel describes how in order to have good sex we need to feel novelty and excitement, as well as security and comfort. She describes it as a dance between an anchor and waves of the ocean. We need a steady and secure relationship with our partner which anchors us to be able to engage in the waves of passion, risk and adventure that we have during sex. The more safe we feel in the relationship, the more comfortable we're going to feel going to risky places with sex.

And we also need to have that security with ourselves. We can't be sexually intimate without also being intimate with ourselves too. To feel physical pleasure, we have to listen to the whims and needs of our body. And for that we need to actually connect with our body. We need to learn to be OK with our nakedness, and we also need to let go of any judgements we hold about our bodies or about sex in general.

Studies show the less confident we feel about our bodies, the more unsatisfying, uncomfortable or boring sex we will have. Some people feel at home in their bodies where others feel at threat or exposed in them. If we feel restricted in our bodies, we'll feel restricted during sex. If we feel shame about our bodies, we will feel shame when being sexually intimate. So the more that we feel assurance and love for the body we come with, the more confident we will feel in initiating and engaging in sexual intimacy with someone we like.

The more comfortable we feel in our bodies, the more comfortable we feel about sex. The more comfortable we feel about being sexual, the better sex we will have.

Real Talk Moment:
- *How do you feel about your body when it comes to sex and sexual intimacy?*
- *What judgements do you hold about sex?*
- *How supportive were your family in helping you understand sex?*
- *Do you remember having 'the talk' about sex? What was that conversation like and how did it shape your views on sex?*

What gets in the way

There are many things that can get in the way of us feeling safe and emotionally present for sexual intimacy. Here are a few:

- Internalized shame about sex: we may have picked up some toxic beliefs about sex from our family, society or from our experiences with sexual partners.
- Internalized shame about our bodies: as we discussed in chapter 10, we might have low confidence about our bodies which can make us critical about them. This can also make us uncomfortable in our own skin, especially when we need to share our body with someone else in such an intimate way.
- Performance anxiety: when we have a perfectionist view about sex or a fear of not being good enough during sex. This might also come from a place of being scared of rejection, where we're worried that our partner will no longer like us after sex.
- Spectatoring: internalized shame, performance anxiety and porn culture can lead us to put all of our focus on how we *look* during sexual activity, which stops us from being in the present moment. It's as though we are watching from a third perspective, instead of allowing ourselves to be present and engaged for potential pleasure.
- Lack of communication about sex: research shows that having open communication about sex can improve sexual intimacy and pleasure. We can do this by having an open dialogue with our partners about what we do and don't like, and debriefing after sex.
- Having poor sexual boundaries: boundaries help us feel safe and secure. When we don't have sexual boundaries on the table, it can make us feel like we have no control over what could happen in the bedroom. If we have non-negotiables,

it's important that we communicate them to whoever we're being sexual with.

- Using sex for the wrong reasons: some people find themselves using sex to numb or distract themselves from their stresses. Whilst sex can be great for relieving our stress, using it as a way to numb ourselves isn't good for us. It often means that we are less present and can also be reliant on sex to solve our problems.

- Using sex to hold a romantic relationship: this can happen a lot in relationships that yo-yo in and out of conflict. In some relationships, sex is used as a reward, punishment or to 'hook someone in'. This might be because we have a warped perception of sex, seeing it only as a way to satisfy our partner and forgetting ourselves in the process. It again stops us from feeling safe, as we hold this massive responsibility of trying to glue the relationship together through sex. Sex is not one person's responsibility, but a collaboration. Also even if a relationship has the most incredible sex, the other elements of the relationship also need to be working.

- Experiences of sexual trauma: if we've experienced sexual violence, sex and sexual pleasure might feel uncomfortable and unsafe. We'll speak more on this later.

- Under the influence: some people cope with their anxieties about sex by having alcohol or drugs beforehand. Whilst this might temporarily cool our nerves, it stops us from being fully present and engaged. To have secure and fulfilling sex, we need to be emotionally present and connected to our bodies.

Do you relate to any of these? What bad sex habits do you have that you might need to let go of? How did they start?

More than just the body

One way to be more sex positive is to understand that sex isn't just about how physically turned on we are. Sexual arousal is about four parts: our brain, our thoughts, our emotions and our body. They all work together in helping us feel aroused and ready for sex. This is called the homeodynamic model of sexuality.

Each of these four parts connect and flow into each other, as if they're having a conversation. They flow into each other to influence how turned on, safe and ready we feel for sex. Imagine it as a group of jurors. For the best outcome, all parts need to unanimously agree that they feel ready for sex.

Brain (tells our thoughts)

Whatever is happening in our body impacts our brain. Our amygdala alarm system will be noticing what feels safe and what doesn't feel safe. And if we're carrying any stress about sex or anything else in our lives, it will show up in our nervous system.

Thoughts (tells our emotions)

Whatever is happening in our brain will impact what's happening in our thoughts. If our amygdala alarm system is relaxed, we might have space for sexy thoughts or fantasies. But if our amygdala is triggered, our thoughts will focus on the stress that we're carrying.

Emotions (tell our body)

Our thoughts impact our feelings. If we're having sexy thoughts, we will feel calm, excitement and playfulness. If our thoughts are anxious, we might feel fear, anger or shame, the unsexiest of emotions which will make us want to pull away from intimacy.

Body (tells our brain)

Our feelings show up as sensations in our body. If we're feeling calm, excited and playful, we'll feel a pleasurable flutter in our stomach. We'll also be open to explore touch from our partner. But if our feelings are fear, anger and shame, any advance from a partner could make our skin crawl.

So whenever you are feeling aroused or not aroused, try checking in with yourself in four ways:

Checking in with your brain

How is my nervous system?
What stress am I carrying?

Checking in with your mind

What thoughts or images do I have and see?
What anxieties/worries are on my mind?

Checking in with your emotions

What emotions am I processing right now?
Are any of these emotions about my partner?

Checking in with your body

What sensations feel sensitive in a good way?
What sensations feel sensitive in a bad way?

Your sex drive

We often talk about sex using a car metaphor: we have high or low sex drive. In her book *Come As You Are*, Emily Nagoski describes Bancroft and Janssen's Dual Control Model. She names a sexual accelerator and sexual brakes which motivate our sex drive.

Our accelerator fires us up for sex by turning us on. It recognizes any smells, sensations or fantasies that inspire us to feel ready and aroused for sexy time. Everyone has different stimuli that will accelerate their sex drive. For some people it might be the feel of lace, or deep meaningful conversation, or the fantasy of a person in uniform. Or it could be all of the above.

Our good sexual experiences inspire our accelerators. Some people have a very sensitive accelerator, which means they have lots of things that arouse them. Others have low-sensitive accelerators, which can mean they might need more time and consideration to get started sexually. Both are normal, and understanding our accelerators is important if we want to feel aroused for sex.

Our brakes cool our sexual drive, or turn us off. Our bad sexual experiences determine these brakes. This includes any turn-offs that we have or any stressful thoughts that we're holding. Like certain colognes/perfumes, being in a messy room or having a lot on your mind. Everyone has different brakes and again it depends on our upbringing and experiences with sex. Again, some people have hyper-sensitive brakes and others might have low-sensitive brakes. Both are normal.

Two people can have very different accelerators and brakes for each other. Something like sexting might be an accelerator for one person, and a major brake for their partner. That's why knowing our accelerators and brakes, as well as our partners, is important for a fulfilling sex life. When this happens, we can use it as an opportunity to have a Real Talk conversation about sex.

Take a moment to reflect on your own drive. You can do this alone, or you might want to do this with a partner too.

What are your accelerators?	What are your brakes?
Things that bring you closer to sex. These can be thoughts, feelings, fantasies, sensations or memories.	*Things that move you away from sex. These can be thoughts, feelings, fantasies, sensations or memories.*
e.g a tidy house, sexting during the day	*e.g. when the neighbours might hear you, work stress*

The wounds of sexual trauma

Our bodies are precious and need to be handled with the tenderness and care that they deserve. But I hear a lot of real-life stories of when people have experienced the opposite. Stories where their bodies were disrespected or violated. I'm talking here about stories of sexual violence.

I wish no one had stories like this, but sadly they exist more frequently than we realize. It is said that over half of women, half of gender-queer people and a third of men have experienced sexual violence. Scarily, one in four of adults have experienced sexual abuse before the age of 18. From child sexual abuse to rape or attempted rape, to coercive sex to elder abuse, sexual violence is an undisputable part of our society. The scar that sexual violence can leave behind can be devastating for the relationship that we have with our bodies and something we need to take a moment to explore. We are about to delve into some difficult waters, so go gently with yourself on these pages. If you need to pause, pause. If you need to skip to a chapter that feels more accessible, do it. But set an intention to return here when you're ready.

Let me start by saying that sexual violence is never our fault. Sadly and wrongly, society has been conditioned to often find fault in the harmed, rather than making the harmers accountable. Most of the time, when someone is sexually harmed it is by someone who knows them in some capacity. Some abusers will have a way of grooming the people they eventually harm by showing how safe and trustworthy they are. This can make it difficult for survivors to heal from this situation and a challenge to work out who is safe and who isn't. But it is never, ever our fault. We did not ask for nor expect what happened.

Sexual violence is so threatening that it can feel close to death, and so our bodies respond by going into freeze mode. Our body shuts down in order to numb us and remove us from the present moment, so that we don't have to live with the pain of it in the here and now. Our fight or flight mode is deactivated, and there is nothing that we can do once this happens. Actress Gabrielle Union described how she saw herself hovering over her own body and empathizing with herself during a rape attack. Our brain and body are simply trying to protect us from the trauma of the present moment. There is nothing we could have done to predict, reverse or change what happened. And if we find ourselves ruminating about it, this is our brain's way of grabbing control of an uncontrollable situation. Sexual violence is never justifiable and our behaviour is never the cause for another person's crimes. So for anyone reading this and holding on to a responsibility that doesn't belong to them, here is a gentle reminder to begin to let go.

Any abuse that is used against us has the power to be traumatizing and life-changing, as described in chapter 5. But sexual violence adds another layer of harm to our bodies and our relationship with sex. It's not uncommon for sexual-trauma survivors to feel betrayed by their bodies after sexual violence. There can be anger at our bodies for freezing, and sometimes for orgasming at a time of such threat (orgasms are a bodily response that do not always equal pleasure). Some survivors start to feel at war with their body rather than in harmony with it. Shame is often the sour aftertaste left behind. Sexual trauma is an act of oppression which passes on wounds of shame. Our bodies might carry the shame of a perpetrator long after they've done what they've done. The shame we carry after sexual trauma often belongs to the perpetrator. By doing what they did, they project their shame onto us.

Body and sexual challenges after sexual violence exist on a spectrum. Our relationship with sex changes. Sex is supposed to be an attachment behaviour that brings us closer. But if sex and sexual contact becomes a weapon used against us, it can block us from sexual pleasure and autonomy.

On the one hand, survivors might find themselves feeling deep aversion, fear and avoidance about sex. This is often called hyposexuality and happens because our amygdala alarm system is triggered by confusing sexual play with the abuse we experienced, and might pull up flashbacks of what we experienced. This slams the brakes on and inhibits our sexual desire and arousal. Every move looks like a red flag to the amygdala, and survivors may find they are distancing themselves sexually and romantically.

On the other hand, some survivors experience a trauma response of hypersexuality and a heightened sex drive. But, like having sex on auto-pilot, this experience of sex can be emotionally barren as, even though our bodies are in it, our minds are dissociated. Hypersexuality from trauma can lead to lots of sexually risky situations such as drunk or high sex, sex with inappropriate partners or unprotected sex. This happens because our amygdala alarm system goes off but instead of avoidance, like hyposexuality, we go into numbing. We unconsciously want to replace the bad feelings with something that might feel good or more within our immediate control: sex. Sex becomes the numbing agent for any residual shame, guilt and fear from what we experienced. So when this happens, what we're really chasing is control over trauma. It can also mean that the need to numb our discomfort overrides trusting our intuition when red flags show up in our sexual relationships.

Another reason why some people go into hypersexuality is because we repeat what we don't repair. When we hold trauma in our bodies that has not been repaired, our body will unconsciously find different ways to re-enact what happened to us. So we find ourselves sexually active in sexually risky situations, and the aftermath is that we are left with new reasons for the same emotions of fear, shame and guilt that we felt after sexual violence. Our body is trying to bring us back to the wound. Like picking at a scab, trying to do over the trauma.

Both of these responses are a natural response to sexual trauma. They show how our body finds different ways to deal with our brain being triggered. The body remembers trauma, so any sensory information relating to sex or how we were harmed will ring a bell for our body to react somehow. And just like any other trauma response, we need to find safety and grounding. To heal our relationship with sex, we need to build a sense of home and healing within our sexuality first.

Healing our relationship with sex

Create a sex-positive vibe

The first thing is learning that sex and sexual abuse are not the same. Sex should be safe, consenting, emotionally close, empowering and fulfilling. Whether we are with a long-term partner or not, sex should be equal, caring and nurturing. Sexual abuse is the opposite in every way. It is unsafe, without consent or consent-coerced, emotionally neglectful, disempowering and traumatizing. As bell hooks says, abuse negates love and care. It's important to know this difference as a reminder that sex is a good thing, not an abusive thing.

If you're dealing with confusing feelings around sex due to past experiences, it might take a little while to let that lesson sink in, but creating a sex-positive mindset will help you find the safety in sex.

- Explore self-pleasure. Self-pleasure is a great way to explore your body, as well as some of your accelerators and brakes. It is about discovering what feels safe and pleasurable, and what doesn't. And whilst we can of course do this with a partner too (please do), the person we might feel safest to explore this with is ourselves.

- Slow down. If the idea of sex is really freaking you out, take it off the table. Share some context as to why, tell your partner that you need a hiatus from sex, and talk about how that would impact you as a couple.

- Safety first. The same way that a driver puts on their seat belt, checks their mirrors and ensures their car is safe to drive, we need to also prioritize our own checks of emotional safety. If we do want to be sexually active, we need to attend to our brakes first. If we're stressed, deal with that first. If we feel frozen by the fear that our neighbours might hear us, put on some music. If we're worried that a family member might walk in mid-sex, schedule a date for when no one is home. And yes, it's OK to schedule sex. Spontaneity in sex isn't only about when we choose to have sex, but also the novelty of how. We need to create a setting where we know our worries have been attended to, so that we can be more present and available.

- Practise mindfulness. Our mind is likely to flutter during sex, and this is especially the case for anyone who has experienced sexual trauma. The brain might be struggling to be present for something that might feel scary and vulnerable. And though we can't control our thoughts, we can practise our capacity to shift away from them. So if a thought does come up whilst doing the do, say hello to it.

Then take a deep breath and patiently tell it you will come back to it later. Focus back on what and who is in front of you. Focus on the sensations on your body. Practising bringing yourself back to the present moment will keep you more present during sex over time. Whatever you practise makes it stronger.

Set boundaries about sex

Sex needs your enthusiastic consent. If your brain, mind, emotions and body don't align towards wanting sexy time, then listen to that. Sadly our society normalizes a loss of power when it comes to sex, especially for women and femmes. Sexual coercion is too normal and too common, leading a lot of people to lose their sexual boundaries because society tells us that our partner has more power in the decision than we do. Or maybe we really love our partner and are worried about rejecting them by saying no to sex. This is likely tied up with childhood wounds of guilt and fear of abandonment and disappointing others.

But the sexiest thing is the power of your boundaries. Gaining clarity over, and communicating, when you do and don't want sex leaves space for desire to grow for you and your partner. Esther Perel says love and desire are not mutually exclusive. You can still love and be attracted to your partner and continue to build those things, whilst still saying no to sex. And having some distance from sex gives room for excitement and fantasy to flourish.

Boundaries around sex would include:

- Asking for and clarifying consent
- Deciding whether you want to have sex
- Deciding whether you feel aroused enough for sex
- Communicating your accelerators and brakes to your sexual partner

- Saying what you do like sexually
- Saying what you don't like sexually
- Communicating what is off-limits
- Having debrief conversations after sex
- Agreeing together about protecting each other's privacy
- Using contraception
- Avoiding alcohol and drugs before sex.

Forgiveness

Lastly, one of the most difficult parts of healing sexual trauma is forgiveness. And for me, forgiveness is not necessarily about forgiving the person that harmed you, because that is a personal decision that you have to make. What's most important is forgiving yourself and forgiving your body.

As I mentioned before, some survivors are angry at their body for how it responded during sexual threat. Some survivors are even angry at their body because they believe it was their body's fault for drawing the attention of the person that harmed them. But let me say it again, it is never our body's fault. All our body did was to exist. And to heal, we need to give it permission to continue to exist free of shame, blame and anger. Forgiveness cuts through the weight of these feelings through self-compassion. It allows us to take flight without shame holding us back.

Shame and blame does nothing for us but keep us stuck. It halts our healing and it poisons our sense of self-love. You might remember my client Grace from chapter 5, who was triggered by the smell of alcohol whilst walking past a group of men. This triggered her amygdala and pulled her into flashbacks of being sexually abused as a child. Lifting shame from her shoulders was a big part of our work together. Slumped in the therapy chair, you could see how much it weighed down her body. But building the bricks of her self-compassion eventually led to her shedding the shame that didn't belong to her.

Self-forgiveness here is about separating the bad feelings we feel from the bad thing that was done to us. It is about shifting the accountability. As my incredible client said 'the shame shouldn't be with me, so I'm not carrying it any more'. Self-forgiveness is a choice.

Exercise: Making Amends with Our Body

Our bodies are capable of so much incredible pleasure, but only if we let them. Here is a grounding exercise to help us reconnect with our bodies, but also to make amends with any shame or judgement we've told our body to carry.

Sit in a comfortable space. Make sure you're warm enough, comfortable enough and present enough. And if you can, close your eyes.

Imagine a light doing a scan over your body, starting at the top of your head and slowly making its way down to other parts of your body. As the warmth of the light slowly travels down, ask yourself the following questions:
What parts of my body do I hold judgement about?
What parts do I feel were not good enough?
What parts do I ignore or neglect?
Do this until you reach the soles of your feet.

Now go back to one particular part of your body which you held judgement for. Allow it to feel the warmth of the light. What does that feel like? What sensations, thoughts or feelings do you have about it?

It's time to give that part a little bit of love. What love did it miss out on? What love did it need? Gently hold, caress or touch that body part if you can. Tell your body something that it has been waiting to hear from you. It could be *I love you, thank you, it's not your fault*. Do you need to apologize to your body for anything?

When you're ready, take a moment to speak to that body part. You might find this easier to do through journaling or writing a note to it.

Ask yourself:

What stories does my body have to tell?

What anger or blame do I hold about this body of mine? If my body could speak, how would it feel about that?

What is missing in this relationship between my body and me?

What can I do every day to give a moment of appreciation to my body going forward?

What boundaries do I need to place with others so as to protect and respect my body?

What boundaries do you need to set for yourself to respect other people's bodies?

Unpacking the shame that you've learned from sex is an important way for us to heal and give self-love to your body. When we let go of any judgements that were fed into our understanding of sex, it opens up space for us to have more sex positivity.

So start to confidently speak about your accelerators and brakes. There is no shame or awkwardness about them. It's OK to say what you want and need, especially when it comes to sexual intimacy. They're important and deserve to be listened to before you give anyone access to the preciousness of your body. And I

hope it unleashes a new layer of pleasure with sex, but also with
yourself.

Dare to fall in love with your body the way you expect a lover to.

Real Talk on Sex

- We internalize societal shame about sex, which impacts how we feel about being sexual.
- The key ingredient for a good sex life is safety with your partner and safety within ourselves.
- How aroused we feel is determined by what is happening in our brain, our thoughts, our emotions and our body. All these parts need to agree with each other.
- Our sexual accelerator gets us turned on; our sexual brakes get us turned off.
- Sexual violence is never our fault and is an incredibly painful trauma to heal from.
- To heal, we need to create a sex-positive environment and sexual boundaries to help us feel safe and liberated.
- We can all benefit from making amends with our body.

12

Identity and Justice

*Sometimes the world we live in doesn't
like it when we show up as our authentic selves.*

One of the best things about the world we live in is also one of its biggest challenges. Our world is gifted with so much diversity. Where we come from, how we look and who we choose to love makes us beautifully unique. There's so much varied experience that we bring to the world.

However, it often also divides us. Sometimes the world we live in doesn't like it when we show up as our authentic selves. And discrimination and privilege influence how smoothly we can move through life.

As a Black woman, it would be impossible for me to write a book without having a chapter dedicated to the ways that oppression makes healing and therapy hard. Wider society is like a home that many of us will feel we don't belong to. So how do we hold on to self-love when the world doesn't love us back? And how do we heal our wounds if the world continues to harm us?

Being 'different'

I grew up and have always lived in London, which is one of the most diverse cities in the world. I grew up surrounded by people who looked like me, but alongside the beauty of other cultures too. But I still had the feeling somehow that I was different and had to behave a certain way to be more socially acceptable. I didn't see many people on television with my complexion or my hair texture or my body shape or size. So I tried what I could to blend in, like straightening my hair or hanging out with the white kids. But the more I tried to lean in to being a socially acceptable Black kid, the more I was moving away from loving myself.

One of the most famous stories about diversity is 'The Ugly Duckling'. A mother duck waited for her eggs to hatch, one by one. After a few days, only one egg remained unhatched and it looked a little different from the others. But eventually it hatched and out sprung a duckling. Except this duckling looked different. His feathers were grey, whilst his siblings' were white. And his beak looked different too. His mother wasn't pleased. Despite the duckling trying his very best to fit in, the other ducklings laughed and called him ugly. He learned to internalize that he was ugly, unwanted and didn't belong because of the way he looked. The ugly duckling wandered off and left his family behind, feeling lonely, sad and rejected.

Many of us may have felt like the ugly duckling in our stories. Our sexuality, race, gender, religion, shape, complexion or hair on our bodies might leave us to feel like the odd ones out. As if our authenticity doesn't fit with the rules of the world. It can feel like an attack on our identity.

This is an experience of 'othering', when someone is treated unfairly because they're seen as different. This type of discrimination means we are dismissed or cast out for our views, values or image not fitting with the majority.

When we're on a journey of healing and self-love, these

experiences of othering or discrimination can set us back ten steps. We can start to question our worth and our value, leaving our confidence to dip. Research shows how people from marginalized groups are more likely to experience anxiety, impostor syndrome, low self-esteem and trauma symptoms.

Just like the parent in the ugly ducking story, the world is a parent who doesn't love all of its children equally. It can feel like we're all on a scale according to our otherness.

> ### Real Talk Moment:
> - *Have you ever felt like an 'ugly duckling' or 'different'?*
> - *How did it feel for you?*
> - *What was it about you or was it the environment you were in that made you feel that?*
> - *Now think of a time when you felt celebrated for who you are. How did it feel? What made you feel that way?*

Privilege and not-privilege

Our social identity is so complex. We can have experiences of privilege because of who we are. But we can also have experiences of what I call not-privilege. For example, white women hold the privileges of being white so they're not likely to be held back by racism, wrongly profiled by the police, or face the ethnicity pay gap. However, being a woman could mean that they face sexism, sexual harassment and the gender pay gap. Privilege and not-privilege can exist at the same time.

We each hold so many different identities. For example, my identities include: being Black, a woman, cisgendered, having a fuller body, working-class upbringing, middle-class lifestyle, masters qualified. Some of these things bring me privilege, and some of these things bring me not-privilege in my everyday life.

One of my favourite tools for showing us our privilege and not-privilege is through the wheel of power (see overleaf, adapted from an image at ccrweb.ca). The wheel of power shows us some of the many different intersectionalities and communities within the Western world.

The groups in the inner circle are those which tend to have more power in society. The groups in the outer circle tend to be marginalized. This means they're more likely to be systematically discriminated against. For example, someone who has significant ADHD would find themselves on the outer circle because most jobs centre around, or assume, neurotypical needs. Job interviews are always stressful, but for someone with ADHD this can be really challenging and might already put them at a disadvantage to their competitors.

Some parts of our identity might be in the inner circle, some might be in the outer circle and some might be in the middle.

So what does power mean? Sometimes I teach workshops to other psychotherapists and this is a tool that I often use to help them think about their privileges and not-privileges. During one of these workshops, someone eagerly leaned forward and put their hand up. By the frown on their face, I could see they were having a hard time with the wheel. They told me they felt like it was an assumption that someone has more power because they're middle-class or educated or a gay man. This person was not happy. I smiled softly and told them I could see where they were coming from. 'Hmm, could you try something, though?' I asked. 'If we swapped the word "power" with the word "safety", would you still disagree?' They looked at the wheel again. I saw the penny drop, before they leaned back in their seat without much else to say. To have safety is powerful. Not to have safety is powerless.

What parts of your identity sit within the outer circle? What parts of your identity sit within the inner circle? What parts of the wheel or your place on the wheel make you feel uncomfortable? When we meet someone for the first time, some parts of the wheel are visible and some parts are

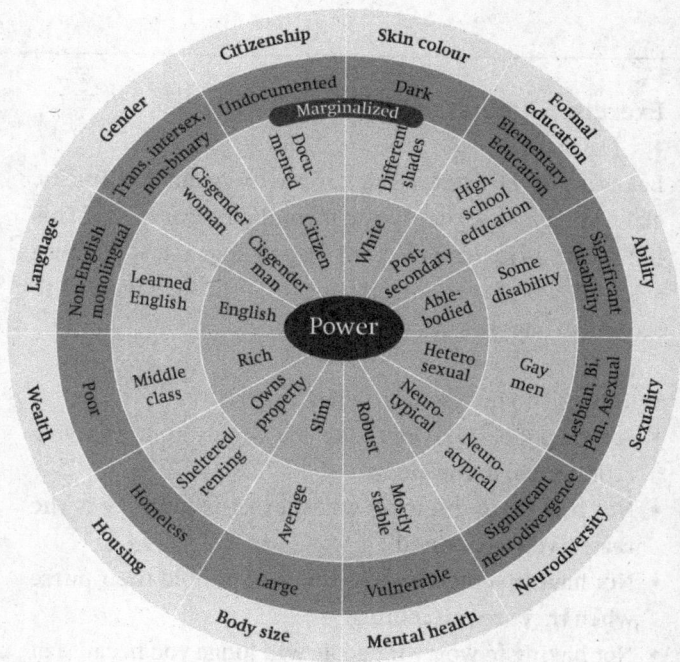

The Wheel of Power: adapted from an image at ccrweb.ca

invisible. What assumptions do people make about you from the way you look?

The social ladder that we exist on is sticky to say the least. So if the wheel of power stirs up some uncomfortable feelings for you, this makes a lot of sense. Stay with it and ask yourself what feelings might be sitting underneath.

Exercise: Understanding Your Privilege

Below is a list of privileges that run across gender, ethnicity, class, language, sexuality and mental/physical ability. This list shows us just how expansive privilege (and therefore safety) can be. Give yourself time to go through this list to see which ones fit your experience.

Signs that you hold some privilege/safety . . .
- Seeing people who look like you widely and positively represented in the media
- Not having to question whether your identity is the reason you were hired
- Not having someone cross the road or hold their purse when they see you coming
- Not having to worry if people will judge you because of your name or how you look
- Knowing someone is dating you for who you are and not because of a kink, fetish or curiosity
- Openly living with your partner
- Not having to use your lived experience as teaching for other people
- Never experiencing impostor syndrome

- Feeling heard and respected when you share your opinion
- Not receiving unsolicited comments about your body
- Having managers or peers in your field who look like you
- Not having to Google how safe a country is before you travel
- Feeling safe to show public displays of affection with your partner
- Not having to text your friends to let them know you got home safely
- Feeling safe and protected by law enforcement
- You received stable education throughout your childhood
- You have a degree
- Having healthy, nutritious food in the kitchen
- Only moving house by choice
- Having parents who can give or lend you money as an adult
- Growing up with parents who could buy you new clothes and toys when needed
- Growing up with family holidays
- Not having to come out about your sexuality or gender
- When your gender is an option on legal forms
- When people know and use your correct pronouns
- Identifying with the gender you were assigned at birth
- Not being questioned about your genitals
- Not needing to use the disabled toilets
- Being white or able to pass as white
- Being colourblind by 'not seeing' race
- Having access to your heritage and family tree
- Having a name people know how to pronounce
- Seeing couples on television that represent your romantic interests

- Never having to conceal your partner or who you choose to love
- Not having to worry about harassment at work or in social spaces
- Being assertive without being called a 'bitch', 'emotional', 'too much' or 'difficult'
- Not being pressured about having children or marriage
- Being able to walk home late at night
- Being sexually empowered without judgement
- Going to new places without worrying about your access needs
- Not feeling pitied by others
- Being able to access most spaces
- Being able-bodied and free from chronic illness
- Not having your accent or dialect mocked
- Not being asked where you're really from
- Finding your clothing size in most stores
- Being neurotypical and never having questioned whether you have neurodiverse needs.
- Never having to navigate racial or queerphobic slurs in your everyday life.

Take a moment to check in with yourself. How did it feel to work through that list? What parts were difficult or surprising?

Safety and self-care

Safety isn't guaranteed to all of us. As a kid, I remember being aware of the murder of Stephen Lawrence, an 18-year-old Black man who was killed during a racist attack whilst waiting for a bus. It took almost twenty years before two of his murderers were convicted, thanks to racism and gatekeeping from the police. I learned from a young age that people who looked like me were not granted safety, even the safety of getting home. All children see the world as safe and fair, until they have their first encounter with receiving or witnessing discrimination that interrupts that view of the world. But if a child isn't from a marginalized community, they might not ever witness or know that discrimination really exists until adulthood, because they've never had to face it. We need safety around us to be able to heal. It's almost impossible to heal when our surroundings can't take care of us.

Self-care isn't always granted to everyone either. My partner is a Black man and we recently spoke about how those of us from marginalized communities don't always have access to the self-care that we need. For example, going on a walk for his mental health in our gentrified neighbourhood costs him more than he gains. He isn't able to relax fully, drop his ego, be himself and have a mindful walk, because his mind is on having to keep up a mask of appearing like the 'good Black neighbour or harmless Black man' to anyone he meets on his walk. He can't even wear a hooded sweater. How wild is it that he has to put his false self on in order to do something for his own wellbeing?

Being seen as different can be difficult for our sense of self-love. I spoke with Alishia McCullough, a mental-health therapist and content creator who specializes in body justice and fat liberation with Queer, Trans, Black, Indigenous, People of Colour (QTBIPOC). During 2020, Alishia became co-founder of the hashtag #AMPLIFYMELANATEDVOICES to lift up the voices and experiences of Black and Brown people. And on its first day, the hashtag had 9,000 posts on Instagram.

Alishia names another way to describe othering: 'body alienation'. She says:

> Body alienation is when you feel that your body is not represented anywhere and that you are completely alone in your experience because your body is so different from everyone else. Sometimes we can even alienate ourselves from our own bodies by leaving them to survive in these environments. I would first encourage folks by saying that your body is not bad, it is not broken. I would also share that it is not your fault for leaving your body to survive, because we have a culture that is invested in you not being in your body so that you can continue to feel as if you don't belong. The first step to coming back into your body is by acknowledging the systemic and cultural traumas that have kept us from being embodied, and then beginning to form a relationship with your body again.

A good ally

Social injustice is a trauma. And so for anyone who is impacted by a social injustice, for example being hurt or seeing someone from their community being hurt for who they are, they're likely to have a trauma response. Just like what we talked about in chapter 7: fight, flight, freeze and fawn.

When these things happen, we need support from good allies to get through. But sometimes allyship can make things worse rather than better. Here are a few examples of unhelpful allyship.

Denial/Fragility: a friend feels uncomfortable and wants to change the topic, so they tell me that I shouldn't be upset and they don't understand why race has anything to do with it. It's likely they are feeling so uncomfortable that they can't bear to be with my reality. This is really dismissive and tones down my experiences of indirect and direct racism.

Guilt: a friend texts to deeply apologize for what happened, to apologize for their part in white supremacy and to apologize for the impact of their privilege. This actually isn't helpful as it would be a responsibility on me to forgive or soothe their guilt.

Entitlement: a friend tells me they want to be a better human being and they need my help to do it. They ask me about my personal experiences of racism. They even ask me to recommend some books and resources for them to read on the topic. Now firstly it's pretty triggering to ask someone to tell you about their traumas . . . especially when it's for your own needs, not theirs. And asking me to educate them about my trauma is completely inappropriate. There is a huge collection of resources out there that we can all have access to if we try.

Tears: a friend who cries in front of me about what had happened because of how upsetting it was. This might sound really empathetic on their behalf, but it's actually pretty dangerous. It puts me in a place to look after their feelings instead of my own, even though what happened directly impacted the community I was from.

Anger: a friend tells me that they're so angry about it that they're going to protest every day this week to show me how much they care. This could be seen as performative. It's amazing that this friend is going to protest, but why do they need to tell me this? Sometimes this can be as a way of trying to prove how good of a human being someone is being, rather than just standing up for what is right without a reward or recognition.

The right way: a friend calls and tells me they are sorry for what is happening in the world. They ask me how I'm feeling and ask how they can support me during this time. They listen without needing anything from me. They don't try to change my feelings or my perspective. They do social-justice work and actively better themselves to inspire change without needing to let me know. This is a good ally.

Healing *through* social justice

Audre Lorde powerfully tells us that caring for ourselves shouldn't be seen as self-indulgent, but as self-preservation and a political act of warfare. When we prioritize our rest and healing, we prioritize ourselves. We remind ourselves of our own worth and value on this earth, that we are going to pause from capitalism and take care of our needs. Alishia tells us that we can find body liberation by 'experiencing freedom within your own body. Even if the systems are still in place, you feel this inner sense of living audaciously, unapologetically, and in alignment with what you were designed to be.'

One of my favourite ways to help myself and my clients heal through social justice is to teach them about the seven types of rest, as designed by Dr Dalton-Smith. Rest is extra-crucial when it comes to trauma and being triggered as it slows down our nervous system and gives us an opportunity to release trauma stored in the body. I've adapted the seven types of rest model to attend to the needs of healing from social injustice, oppression, othering and trauma.

Physical rest
- Good sleep hygiene
- Naps
- Physical activity to energize your body
- Physical activity to release stored-up cortisol

Mental rest
- Having good work boundaries
- Booking time off
- Resting your mind outside of work

Emotional rest
- Being with people who you can be your real authentic self with
- Having someone to offload your emotions with
- Finding a therapist who has a similar intersectionality

Social rest
- Allowing yourself to take up space
- Avoiding spaces that require you to be a lesser, diluted version of yourself
- Going where you are loved, celebrated and seen (including your job)
- Letting go of friendships that don't genuinely see you

Creative rest
- Finding beauty and inspiration around you, such as connecting with your heritage and identity
- Stepping into nature for inspiration and peace
- Releasing shame through creativity

Sensory rest
- Taking time away from devices
- Setting boundaries around triggering content like the news or traumatic content, and seeking out joyful content
- Allowing silence

Spiritual rest
- Reconnecting with your sense of purpose and belonging
- Connecting with or supporting your community
- Finding inspiration from your faith, prayer or meditation.

Exercise: Loving on Your Identity

Our identity should always be a beautiful part of us. Who we are is never a problem. It's the world around us that has its issues. Everyone is deserving of safety, self-worth and self-love. It's our birthright.

Write a short, sweet love letter to a community you belong to. You might belong to many communities and want to write a love letter to each. Write it and read it out to yourself. It's also important to ask yourself how connected you feel to your community. This might be a sign to find more ways of meeting people who have a similar lived experience to you through community groups and events.

Now, write a longer love letter to yourself and your intersectionality. Reflect on what you love about being authentically yourself, what you love about being a part of your community and how it feels to be around people who look or feel like you.

Real Talk on Identity and Justice

- Many of us may have felt like the ugly duckling in our stories because of our identity (e.g. sexuality, race, gender, religion, etc.).
- We might be othered if our authenticity doesn't fit with the norms of the world.
- We all hold privilege and not-privilege. Both can exist at the same time.
- How safe we feel is a big sign of how much privilege or power we hold.
- When we prioritize our rest and healing, we prioritize ourselves.

13

The Ups and Downs of Stress

Burnout is not a badge of honour.

Life is full of ups and downs and it can be as unpredictable as a game of snakes and ladders. There will be obstacles and challenges to trip us up. But there will also be pivotal moments that help us rise again. And whilst we do our best to move with the ebb and flow of life, just like the weather, our mood is constantly changing. Mood is the weather we have to walk in, whether that be delicious sunshine or heavy rainfall. It changes the ease with which we move through life in that moment. As human beings, how we feel changes with the winds of what we go through. But just as no weather lasts for ever, no mood lasts for ever either. Eventually a new day breaks and it passes on to the next.

In therapy, I hear people hold expectations of their own mood all the time. They say that they're being too dramatic or too emotional or too moody. Or they apologize for crying, ranting or bragging. But these are forms of human expression that deserve to be given the spotlight.

The sooner we realize that we can't always be at our best, the sooner we forgive ourselves and show self-love. Chronic stress and experiences like grief and loss leave us with burdens to carry as we navigate life. We are just human beings doing the best we can with the feelings we have and the weight we have to carry. We are not defined by what we feel. We can only hold it until it passes.

Let's talk about stress

When someone asks us how we are, how often do we say more about how stressed we are instead of how we're *actually* feeling? That's because stress is often the centrepoint of our mood. The same way the flow of water changes depending on the pressure put on it, the flow of how we feel changes when there's the pressure of stress on our shoulders.

Stress is the mental or emotional tension we feel from holding some demanding circumstances. If mood is the weather we have to walk in, stress is the baggage we have to carry. How much we are carrying emotionally or mentally at one time influences how we feel and our capacity to feel.

What is stressful for one person might not feel as stressful to someone else. This isn't necessarily about *what* we're carrying but *how long* we are carrying that stress for. Picture picking up a glass of water and holding it up in front of you at eye level. Whether the glass is half-empty or full, the weight would be pretty tolerable at first. But after a couple of minutes, our arm may start to quiver. After an hour, our arm would probably go numb and be in recovery for the rest of the day. The same thing is true for stress. How long we hold stress for is what makes it most difficult. How long we have been holding stress for in our life story matters. Some people are holding stress for years, maybe even generations, as we've talked about before. Some people have to carry stress wherever they go thanks to the stress of discrimination, where they have additional challenges due to who they are and what they look like, as we covered in chapter 12.

By the way, stress isn't necessarily a bad thing. The whole

purpose of stress is to motivate our bodies into action so we can run from predators and threats. Centuries ago, the predators causing a threat were lions, tigers and bears. But for us now, our predators are modern-day anxieties like our jobs, moving house, interpersonal conflict or even our inner critic. Whether it's a big bear or a scary boss, our nervous system responds in the same way. It impacts our vagus, a collection of nerves which connect our brain, nervous system and gut. Stress sparks a set of reactions in these parts of our body to prepare and get us through the stressor ahead.

To understand when stress is *too much*, we can learn from the Window of Tolerance.

According to psychiatrist Dan Siegel, we all have a window of tolerance. Let's imagine it as a thermometer. At the centre of the thermometer, we have our ideal temperature. This is our window of tolerance and it represents our ideal and optimum levels of arousal and stress. In other words, our emotional capacity. But outside of that window, we have hyper-arousal at the top and hypo-arousal at the bottom of the thermometer.

When we are within our window of tolerance, we are at our emotional best. We feel our most present and connected which means we can reach joy, creativity, laughter and love. We're able to feel like the best versions of ourselves because we're at our most safe and relaxed, our ideal temperature. But when stress becomes too much, our emotional capacity gets maxed out and we have to leave our window of tolerance. Instead we move into hyper-arousal or hypo-arousal.

When we're in hyper-arousal, all the stress we're carrying makes us feel panic, anxiety and frustration. Our heartbeat increases because our body goes into fight or flight mode and it can be pretty overwhelming. It can feel like things are chaotic and out of our control. Its like we're on the hot end of the thermometer.

When we're in hypo-arousal, we've been carrying stress for

so long that we start to feel disconnected, numb and hopeless.
Our heartbeat slows down as our body is so overwhelmed from
carrying stress that it shuts itself down. It can feel like we're on
auto-pilot. We're the cold end of the thermometer and existing at
our bare minimum.

Hyper-arousal and hypo-arousal are not comfortable spots to
be in. So when we do catch ourselves there, we need to find ways
to come back to our window of tolerance. But that can be a lot
easier said than done, since we can get caught up in a cycle of stress
before we even get a chance.

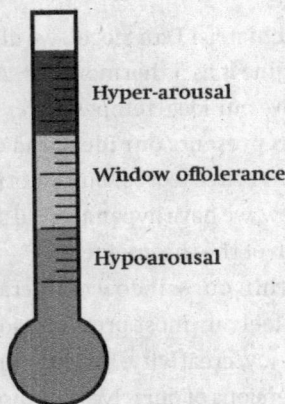

Hyper-arousal

Window of tolerance

Hypoarousal

Real Talk Moment:

- *How stressed have you been feeling lately?*
- *What kind of things tend to cause you stress?*
- *What would someone notice about you and the way you
  are when you're stressed?*
- *What stresses have you been carrying for a long time?*

The stress cycle

I hate the word 'lazy'. It's a word that is often thrown about and in
a judgemental way. We use it to describe when we are unwilling or

unmotivated. But, Real Talk, are we lazy or are we recovering from being in a constant cycle of stress?

Stress is something that we can't always avoid, but our body needs to go through this motion and find a way to complete the process, without getting stuck in the loop of a stress cycle. The stress response cycle is broken into three parts:

- **Alarm**. Alarm is when we're in a hyper-arousal state. The amygdala alarm system in our brain notices that we are at threat and moves our body into survival mode, ready for battle. It triggers our fight-or-flight response and releases adrenaline and cortisol (stress hormone). This increases our blood-sugar levels, heartbeat and energy so that we can fight or run away from our stress, aka our big bear or scary boss.

- **Resistance**. After a while, the stressful thing isn't so stressful any more, so our body slows down to recover. When the stressful event is over, our heartbeat slows down and our cortisol levels reduce. Our body starts to repair itself, but it still stays alert until the stressor is fully over. It's like our body is resting whilst keeping one eye open. The problem is that modern-day stress is a lot more complicated than it used to be. A big bear can be killed and no longer be a threat, but a scary boss isn't going anywhere. This type of stressor is chronic and leaves our body hypervigilant and keeps cortisol running through our veins. Our body adapts to deal with higher levels of stress than it should deal with. This often leads to sleep troubles, poor concentration and crankiness. If the stressful thing is over, our body recovers and goes back to rest mode. But if the stressful thing continues to be an issue, our body goes back to alarm. Rinse and repeat.

- **Exhaustion**. Eventually our body gets bored and tired of going back and forth from alarm to resistance and back again. Staying in the resistance stage for too long is so exhausting for us and our bodies that it leads to burnout, fatigue, anxiety and depression. Cortisol stored in our bodies weakens our immune system, so we'll be more likely to become physically ill too.

Exhaustion is when we're in a hypo-arousal state, i.e. we have no energy. But because so many of us don't realize that is what's happening, we label ourselves lazy instead. In reality, we could be in a constant state of exhaustion if we're always having to fight off stressful things.

When stressors won't stop coming our way or when we haven't recovered from our last stressor, we get stuck in the loop. Some of us might even be so familiar with being in a stress cycle that we become hooked on the feeling of being stressed all of the time. It has become our norm. And childhood has a big part to play with this too. Research shows how having a stressful childhood leads our body to become desensitized or oversensitized to the cortisol in our bodies.

Signs of burnout

Burnout happens when our stress has reached exhaustion level. It's when we've exceeded our capacity and are running on survival mode. Our mind and body are running on limited energy, leading us to have a limited mental, emotional and physical capacity.

Burnout is not a badge of honour. Our body is shutting down and desperately asking us to rest.

Signs of burnout can show up as . . .

- Feeling low and critical all of the time
- Avoidance, anxiety or dread
- Difficulty concentrating
- Difficulty with sleeping and eating habits
- Constantly tired

- Anger, frustration or resentment
- Feeling emotionally numb
- Headaches
- Stressful dreams or nightmares
- Wobbly boundaries
- Daydreaming or dissociating
- Getting physically ill a lot
- Difficulty with intimacy
- Neglecting our emotional needs.

> **Real Talk Moment:**
> - *How does your body tell you when you're burned out?*
> - *What keeps you in burnout mode?*
> - *What things can you do to prevent getting to burnout stage?*

Wild thoughts

Stress doesn't just impact our body and our energy, it also takes its toll on our mind. We can find ourselves having some pretty wild and negative thoughts when we're stressed. It's like we suddenly have a dark cloud over our heads, where everything we see is through a negative filter. Stress attracts more stress, and so we find ourselves with more things to worry obsessively about. What we pay attention to grows. Our inner critic is more likely to be in control and our thoughts feel more hyper-critical, self-blaming, judgemental and closed-minded.

This is because stress stops us from reaching our upstairs brain, our prefrontal cortex, where our capacity for reflection and self-compassion lives. It's like when our mobile phone is in battery-saver mode and working on limited functioning for self-preservation.

When our brain is in battery-saver mode, the thoughts that we pay most attention to are also the most unhelpful ones. These look like:

Catastrophizing. Our thoughts ask 'what if . . .?' and take us to the worst-case scenario. *e.g. What if something bad happens to my family?*

Overgeneralizing. Our thoughts make generalized conclusions and apply them to all situations. *e.g. My whole life is a mess.*

Emotional reasoning. Our thoughts use our emotions as facts. *e.g. I know something bad is about to happen because I can feel it.*

Magnification. Our thoughts exaggerate our imperfections and errors. *e.g. I ruined the whole relationship.*

Minimalizing. Our thoughts minimize our own qualities. *e.g. They said I did a good job but they say that to everyone.*

All-or-nothing thinking. When our thoughts tell us that everything is either wrong or right, bad or good. *e.g. I gave her so much support and she gave me nothing.*

Personalization. When our thoughts tell us that we have to take all of the blame and responsibility. *e.g. It's my fault that my parents are breaking up.*

Mind reading. When our thoughts assume that we know how someone is going to react to us. *e.g. OMG, they're going to hate me.*

Predictive thinking. When our thoughts decide that we can predict the future. *e.g. I'm gonna fail.*

Should/Must. When our thoughts put unrealistic expectations on ourselves or other people. e.g. *I should stay up all night to finish this.*

These unhelpful thinking patterns are manifestations of our triggered amygdala alarm system. We are stuck in alarm mode and we can't help but see more danger ahead. Our alarm system has been so familiar with the stress cycle that it becomes over-sensitized to threat. And our thoughts distort themselves to fit the narrative that we are in continued danger. It also helps to continue the cycle of stress, as our inner critic becomes another stressor to keep us on a loop.

When we're stressed, we also revert back to the ways we coped with stress as children. This includes blaming ourselves, shutting down and isolating ourselves or taking care of the needs of other people. These unhelpful thinking patterns can often be deep-rooted. But one way that we can challenge them is to question their substance. What proof do these thoughts have? What evidence suggests that they are right? What evidence suggests they are wrong? Where are the receipts? Taking a step back to evaluate whether these thoughts are substantial or just our amygdala acting up can be a great way to gain perspective and rebalance our mindset.

Real Talk Moment:

- *What unhelpful thinking patterns do you see in yourself?*
- *What might be helpful to tell yourself when that thought surfaces again? If you're unsure, talk about it with someone you trust to see if they can help.*

Breaking the stress cycle

Stress is something we all go through and what makes it most challenging is that we can lose ourselves whilst we're feeling it. It clouds our capacity for self-love and it can interrupt our healing process too. The more stressed we are, the less access we have to our self-care resources. If only we could get to these resources, they would actually make us feel less stressed. It's like driving round and round on a roundabout, where we have to take an exit to get off it. The only thing that can disrupt us from repeatedly going around our stress cycle is to find a road that's going to change the path of stress remaining in our bodies. We need stress cycle-breakers, acts of self-care, that help our body recover from stress.

We can imagine cycle-breakers as roads that can lead us off the roundabout. They take us away from the repetitive sequence of alarm, resistance and exhaustion. Instead, we can exit the roundabout and take a road that brings us safety, social connection and rest, via a slip road called the ventral vagal. This road slows down our nervous system so we can move from our sympathetic nervous system (fight or flight) to our parasympathetic nervous system (rest and digest). By doing this, we tell our bodies *It's OK, we made it! We survived the big bear. We're safe now.* Here are some scientifically proven ways to break your own stress cycle:

Shake the nerves off

Animals in the wild go through stress cycles all of the time. Like gazelle in the Serengeti who have to run for their lives most days to escape cheetahs and wild dogs. Once they have escaped, they do this funny thing . . . they shake. They shake their head, their torso and every limb of their body before continuing on with their day. You might notice this if you own a dog too. Animals shake after moments of intense stress because it helps them to release adrenaline and cortisol stored in the body. In other words, they are releasing all of the tension and stress so they can return back to a relaxed state. They are literally shaking the nerves off.

As humans, we can take a leaf out of their book by shaking too. You might start by shaking your wrists. Work your way up, shaking the full length of your arms. Then your torso, head and shoulders. And finally your legs. It might feel a little weird at first, so play some upbeat music to help you along. Another way to release cortisol in the body is stretching our limbs, which is why yoga is so great for stress and trauma. Take time stretching each part of your body, giving special TLC to any parts that feel tense or stiff (the neck and shoulders are magnets for stored cortisol).

Trick the cycle

Another way to break our stress cycle is to trick it by tiring it out. As we know, stress makes our brain send more adrenaline and cortisol into our body, as if we are about to run from a big bear. Most of the time, though, the stressors we deal with today don't involve us being as active as that. So we have these energetic hormones in our body that don't really have anywhere to go. Doing cardio exercise like going for a run, exercise class or boxing is a great way to imitate how we would run from a big bear and use up these hormones. It also tires our body, so that our nervous system is more likely to get itself off the roundabout of alarm and resistance.

Body scans and meditation

A body-scan meditation like the one we learned in chapter 11 is great for slowing down our nervous system. When we're stressed, we focus our attention on being hypervigilant to what is happening in front of us and outside of our bodies. This usually makes us more stressed since we'll probably notice even more things to be stressed about as our brains enjoy a negative feedback loop. Body scans are a type of interoception, where we turn our attention inward for our body to remind us that we actually are safe . . . A scary boss isn't actually as life-threatening as a big bear. It can also help to slow down our heart rate, forcing our body into rest and digest mode.

Permission to cry

Have you ever felt better after a cry? Yep, there's a reason for that. When we cry, our body releases endorphins, an internal opiod. This is literally our body's natural supply of a painkiller, which relieves our physical and emotional pain. So if you feel pent-up energy like frustration or sadness, it might be time to make space for your tears. Allow yourself to sit with the vulnerable feelings waiting to surface. Or if your tears feel stuck, cuddle up to a hot-water bottle on your chest whilst watching a movie that you know usually taps your tender spots.

Love hormones

Usually when we're stressed, the last thing we want to do is to make bids for connection and affection. Stress usually shuts our social capacity down, which is why we become more irritable and cranky. But genuine social connection is a great exit road off the roundabout because it takes us straight back to safety. Being heard, hugged or having our hand held creates oxytocin, a love hormone which naturally reduces cortisol.

Sleep and rest

Sleep is good for our wellbeing. Getting eight-plus hours of sleep every night allows our body time to recover from carrying stress in the day. Create a routine where you allow time to unwind before bed and gently rise in the morning. Also remember that light from screen time before bed keeps our fight-or-flight system activated, so shut it down at least an hour before sleep.

Exercise: Stress Cup of Tea

Imagine that you can measure your stress levels as a cup of tea. The more stressed you feel, the emptier your cup is. The less stressed you feel, the fuller your cup is.
How do you know when your cup is full?
What is something you can do for yourself when your cup feels empty?
What is something you can do for yourself when your cup feels completely empty?

Write it down and share it with someone who is likely to be around you when you're stressed. They can encourage you to tap into these things.

Let me say that all of these are easier said than done. It can be really hard to reach for our stress-cycle-breakers when we're stressed and so a lot of us can get frustrated with ourselves in hindsight, once we do feel more regulated. *Why didn't I ask for help when I was so stressed?* Or, *It's so obvious to me, I should have . . ., it probably would have made me feel better sooner.* When we are at peak stress levels, we often have our blinkers on. All we can see is our stressor. It consumes our thoughts, feelings and fears, and its stress response consumes our bodies. It's only once the stressor has passed and we're feeling calmer that we realize *Oh yeah, I could have tried that thing!*

It can also be hard to motivate ourselves to do these things once we are in alarm, resistance and especially exhaustion. A lot of the time, self-care is about choosing to do things that we need to do for the long-term, rather than what we want to do in that moment.

So ask yourself, what will be best for Future Me? Something that can be helpful for this is making these cycle-breakers a part of our regular routine, rather than quick fixes for your mental health. Also sharing these cycle-breakers with your loved ones means that they can offer them up to you once they see you stuck in alarm, resistance or exhaustion.

Real Talk on the Ups and Downs of Stress

- Stress is the tension we feel from carrying some demanding circumstances.
- What you experience as stressful might not be as stressful to someone else. It's not about *what* we're carrying but *how long* we are carrying it for.
- Stress moves in a cycle until we find space to recover: alarm, resistance and exhaustion.
- Burnout is when our body is shutting down from exhaustion and desperately asking us to rest.
- Our inner critic is in full control when we're stressed, leading to more unhelpful thinking patterns.
- We need acts of self-care which can break the stress cycle to help us recover.

14

Grief

Grief is the price that we pay for how deeply we loved.

We thrive with healthy attachments, so what about when we have to lose them? Loss is one of our biggest fears, but also our most inevitable pains. And since we thrive on constancy, connection and attachment as humans, grief can be something that we have no idea how to deal with.

But it's not just us. Our culture has an avoidant attachment with grief and death. We've been taught to use euphemisms like 'passed away' to soften the blow of talking about death. We've been shut down to stop talking about our loss once the funeral is over. And we forget to ask questions like *Tell me about the person you lost?* As a result, so many of us have to carry our grief in silence. The person that we lost becomes He-who-shall-not-be-named yet who we are so longing to talk about. Carrying their memory and the pain their absence leaves us can be one of the loneliest experiences many of us will face. The weight of it carries a burden on our mood and obstructs us from healing through our grief.

Misconceptions about grief

Because of the way that culture deals with loss and grief, there are many toxic assumptions about grief which stand in the way of our permission to go through it. Here are some of those misconceptions and the Real Talk that we can hold on to instead.

#1 Grief is about death

Grief has often been thought of as the deep sorrow and loss after a person has died. But we're becoming more aware that grief isn't just about the death of a loved one.

Ironically, our first-ever experience of grief is our own birth. As babies in the womb, we are in complete bliss. We have everything we will ever need: warmth, nurture, nourishment and being as intimate with our birth parent as we'll ever be. Until suddenly, our homely womb pushes us out and into a strange, less holding world. So as newborn babies, we grieve our first home, the womb. Why am I telling you this? Because this first universal experience of grief gets resurfaced whenever we feel loss later on in our life. But it's so unconscious and pre-verbal that most of us won't know, though we will feel it. When we lose someone we love as children or adults, it takes us to our earliest inner-child wound of being taken away from comfort and safety.

Grief is a natural human response to the loss of a loved person, animal, object or life transition. It is the sorrow that we feel when we have come to the end of a chapter in our lives that we can never go back to. Grief is about any type of loss, including:

- a miscarriage
- loss of a relationship or friendship
- loss of health (e.g. if someone were diagnosed with cancer)
- loss of a job or financial stability
- loss of a pet
- loss of our childhood or the childhood we should have had

- loss of safety after trauma
- loss of a dream or goal
- loss of freedom or autonomy
- moving home.

Many of these things trigger our grief because we are grieving the end of a relationship or a sense of safety. Whatever the reason for our loss, it's important that we validate it rather than shut down the feeling. There is no wrong or right thing deserving of our grief.

> **Real Talk Moment:**
> - *Take a moment to reflect on your experience of grief. What experiences of grief did you have as a child?*
> - *Who was there to help you make sense of it?*
> - *And what experiences of grief have you had as an adult?*
> - *Were you able to make space for your grief?*

#2 Grief is just sadness
Grief is more than just sadness. And though emotions are one part of our grief, it also shows up in other ways too. For example, grief can have a physical impact on us. Grief can bring us anxiety, nightmares, digestive problems, body pains and weight loss or weight gain.

Some of us might feel guilt. Loss can remind us that life is too short and too unpredictable. So our ego grasps for control in the form of guilt. This type of guilt is when a part of us blames ourselves for contributing to losing them or not making enough time for the relationship with them when they were present. It puts a heavy burden on us and stands in the way of processing our sadness and tapping into how loved we were. Grief is a symbol of our love. It is how we love them after they have gone and how we preserve that relationship without them being close to us.

But we don't have a time machine and we can't go back in time. We have no magic wand to help us change things. Falling into a hole of self-criticism doesn't help us. When this happens, we can try to imagine speaking to our loved one about it. What would they say about the situation? If they could witness your guilt, what words would they say to you? If it's helpful, hold on to this and repeat it to yourself. If it's hurtful, find some words of wisdom from someone else with a kinder outlook, like your Fairy Godmother from chapter 7.

Some of us might feel anger. It's natural to feel anger at the unfairness of loss. Without our control, something or someone we cherished is gone. And they're not even here for us to tell them how angry we are with them for leaving. That anger has nowhere to go. Sometimes it gets projected onto other people. We might push people away or have a short fuse. But a lot of the time, if that anger isn't given a safe outlet, we internalize it. We direct those angry feelings back to ourselves in the form of guilt. We look back and criticize our past memories with our lost one; we reprimand ourselves for not being good enough or present enough or appreciative enough; our magical thinking might have us imagining how things might have unfolded differently if we had acted differently. But your grief needs your kindness.

#3 We grieve in stages

Thanks to Kübler-Ross's Five Stages of Grief, many people assume that grief has an order to it. The five stages tell us that we usually feel:

Denial – 'I'm fine' or 'This doesn't feel real'
Anger – 'Leave me alone' or 'I hate them for leaving me'
Bargaining – 'I'll do anything to bring them back'
Depression – 'What's the point in being here?'
Acceptance – 'It hurts, but I'm going to be OK'

The truth is, grief is messy as hell. Yes, there are different parts to it, like acceptance, denial and anger. But there is no sequence and we can re-grieve over and over again. The journey of grief is more messy and weird than it is neat and linear. There can be an expectation to move through stages of grief in order to move on with the rest of our lives. But we don't have to and shouldn't have to 'move on' from our loved one. That's a societal expectation.

Just like other painful experiences, grief changes us. In *The Order of the Phoenix*, Harry Potter realizes he can see a horse-like creature, Thestrals, that no one else can see. Actually, the only people who can see them are other people who have seen death. Everyone else remains oblivious to their existence. This is a little of what happens for those of us who go through loss. We start to see the world differently and there's a different awareness and insight on life. This is called 'situatedness', and is when our life experiences and where we are situated in life impact how we see and live in the world. For example, after losing a loved one, the way that we see Christmas and birthdays might change because now we have to experience those days without their presence.

#4 Grief is about saying goodbye and moving on
Grief isn't about saying goodbye or getting closure, that's a Western expectation. In lots of non-Western cultures, bereavement is honoured through a celebration of life and connecting to our lost ones. For example, in my British–Jamaican culture, funerals are a celebration of life. An experience of coming together to eat, drink, dance and roar with laughter as we grieve through joyous stories.

Grief is also an ongoing process of actually staying close to our loved one, even when they're no longer there. In Continued Bonds theory, Klass, Silverman and Nickman believe that we can't leave our loved ones behind, instead we need to carry their memory along with us. We can do this through talking about them, continuing rituals connected with them, and bringing the values and sentiment of our relationship with them to keep them in our lives. Despite what we've been made to think, holding on to a loved one is allowed and healthy as long as we can also be present to the rest of our lives and connections.

Do you remember in *The Lion King* when Simba sees his father's face in his own reflection? And when Rafiki laughs and says 'He lives in you'? We internalize our loved one, and that internalized version of them lives within us. So that even decades later they grow with us. Continued bonds can help us in healing our grief and facing our future fears and challenges. For example, I've had clients who lost parents in childhood. When they've needed solace and parental guidance in solving adult challenges, they've found themselves imagining what advice would mum or dad give if they were here.

In therapy, it's rare for my clients to wish they could move on from their grief. Instead, it's more common that they ask to make more space for the person they're grieving. We want a space to remember and to say their names aloud, to allow them to exist where other parts of our life may have tried to forget who we are grieving. We live in 'move on' culture, where it's not OK to dwell or linger on things from the past. Including people from our past. But what if those people brought us love, joy or comfort? And even if they brought us pain, we can't say goodbye to whole chapters of our story just because a character had to make an unplanned exit.

> When Dylan's mother died suddenly, she left behind his broken heart. She was a reserved woman, so Dylan felt like he was grieving a parent he didn't have the chance to know as a person. There were so many questions he never had the chance to ask her.
>
> I asked Dylan whether there were any other ways for him to feel connected with her, and he soon discovered her entire collection of vinyl records. Through listening to

her musical tastes, he felt more connected to her than he could ever remember. Listening to these vinyls allowed him to get to know her outside of being just his quiet, reserved mum. Though some of her records raised more questions (Wtf, Mum? I didn't know you listened to Led Zeppelin!?), it made him feel more connected to her than he had ever felt before, as he was discovering new parts of her. He also began to take a new interest in vinyl records, and going to vinyl record stores became a new pastime for him where he could keep his mother in mind along the journey. Even playing one of her most treasured vinyl records at his wedding when the opportunity came. Music became a way of saying goodbye, but also finding a way to carry his mother's presence with him as his life continues.

I believe it's important that we keep a sense of connection and conversation with our loved one. I once saw an article which said there are cemeteries around the UK with postboxes to mail letters to our loved ones. I love this idea of posting letters to our loved ones when we want to feel close to them.

Music is also so powerful in holding powerful memories and emotions for us in just a few minutes of song. I often encourage my clients to create a music playlist full of songs that remind them of their loved one, which they can access whenever they miss them or need to feel close to them. A soundtrack to the relationship we had and will continue to have with them.

#5 Grief gets easier, the first year is the hardest

Grief is one of the hardest experiences that we will go through in life. It is also the most inevitable experience of trauma that we will go through in life. But grief has no expiry date. There is no deadline by which we will have done with our grief.

The first year can be tough, but so can the anniversaries that follow. Even if we don't notice it on a conscious level, we might find ourselves with a rush of emotion when the time draws near because our body remembers.

#6 All grief is the same

It's also important to say that the more complicated the relationship, the more complicated the grief. Grief is always hard, but some experiences can be more complex than others. These include:

- Losing someone we were estranged from or no longer spoke to
- Anticipatory grief (for example terminal or progressive illness)
- Losing a baby through birth trauma, miscarriage or abortion
- Losing someone to suicide
- Not being able to attend the funeral or other rituals.

Complicated grief like losing a loved one to suicide or losing someone after estrangement is so tough. In my experience, when this happens we are left with so many unresolved feelings, thoughts and questions. Any feelings of shame, guilt, fear, regret, loneliness and despair that were left behind by the person who died get reclaimed by their friends and family. Especially because there is still so much societal shame about suicide or estrangement from family. And when we've lost someone in that way, it can leave us with regrets and questions. Give yourself grace and know that your love continues on through your mourning and remembering all of who they were, not just how they died.

> *Shanice had always been close to her father. But she was 12 years old when he died by suicide. Understandably, his death was a shock for Shanice and her family. And they dealt with it in the only way that they knew how*

to: getting on with things. They never cried together
and hardly ever spoke about her dad and his absence.
Shanice herself boxed up all her feelings and memories
of Dad as the rest of her life moved on. She completed
her school education uninterrupted and went to college.
When she made it to university, her life felt really dark
and she found herself having her own thoughts about
taking her life. She was carrying the emotional burdens
that he had left behind.

In therapy, we opened space to talk about her dad
every day. Bringing to life things that he would say and
do, and how some of his most adorable quirks were the
same as Shanice's own. We had to remember that even
though he wasn't here physically, he was still a part of
her life. And to unlock how the shame she felt about how
he died was blocking her access to him so that she could
mourn and stay connected and alive with his memory.

#7 Grief is easier when you're a child

I've learned that people disregard their grief because they
experienced it in their childhood. Children are often forgotten
when it comes to grief. Grown-ups assume that children don't fully
understand what's going on and so they're often left out of the
conversation. They might even not get a chance to go to the funeral
of their loved one, because grown-ups want to keep them away
from death.

No matter how old we are, we feel grief. Whether we are one year
old or one hundred years old, the loss of a important connection can
be a blow. As children, we might not always have the language for
it, though, which makes it even more complicated to grieve.

Something that helps with my clients who have lost parents
or siblings at a young age is reminding them that we grieve
over and over again. As we go through different life stages and

milestones, we're reminded that the person is no longer with us. There can also be a feeling of: I wish they knew me as I am now. And this opens up an opportunity to be with our grieving feelings again, and to heal on a deeper level than we did before. Grief isn't linear and it doesn't disappear. Instead, our life grows bigger around it, until it no longer feels like the biggest thing in our life.

Exercise: Collecting Memories

A fear that many of us have when we've lost someone we love is whether we will also lose our memory of them. We want to soak up and remember every single detail of them so that we can hold them in mind for ever. Remembering their scent, their laugh or their quirks is a great way to keep their memory alive within us.

One way of capturing this is through a memory box or jar. This involves collecting photographs, belongings, notes connected to the person we loved and lost and placing them in a safe container that you can access whenever you need to. The idea is that you have a time capsule of sentimental items which take you back to your memory of them whenever you feel it starting to slip. Sometimes we don't have any objects that we can use, so we can also write and add notes or letters too. On a sad and difficult day, it might be an idea to write a note to add to the box. Here are a few prompts of what you could write when you're ready to slowly add to your memory box:

Describe your favourite memory with your person
Describe your earliest memory with your person

Describe your last memory with your person
What did your person smell like?
How did your person greet you? Did they have any nicknames for you?
How did your person dress? Did you have a favourite outfit?
What do you hope your person knows about you?
What things did your person do to express their love for you?
What do you wish you could say to your person?
What do you know about your person's childhood?
Are there any stories or jokes that your person told you that you'd like to hold on to?

Grief is the price that we pay for how deeply we loved. And though it aches and breaks our heart, it's also validation that we experienced something that was special and big which we can internalize and carry with us for the rest of our lives. As Winnie the Pooh says, how lucky we are to have had something so hard to say goodbye to.

Writer Arthur Golden describes grief like a window that suddenly opens without our permission. The room goes cold and we get a chill, and we're left in a feeling of cold stuckness. It chills every part of us, making it hard to get moving again. But slowly the window opens a little less each time and we might even forget that it's there. Until one day when we realize we don't feel so cold any more.

Real Talk on Grief

- Western culture is pretty avoidant about talking about grief or death, which can make it a difficult environment to heal.
- Grief isn't only about the death of a loved one, but also could be about an animal, object or life transition.
- Grief can be messy as hell and we don't need to do it in stages.
- We don't need to move on. It can be helpful for our healing to find ways to still feel connected to who or what we lost.

15

Trying Therapy

When life give you lemons, try therapy.

After I trained to be a psychotherapist, there was one question people in my personal life kept asking: how do I approach therapy? I realized that so many people wanted to invest in their mental wellbeing and healing through therapy, but had no idea where to start. More people were realizing that it's OK not to be OK, and it's also OK to look for help.

Healing and our self-love journey can be like learning to swim. It's safe enough for us to waddle in the shallow end alone when the water just about reaches our waist. However, when it comes to learning how to swim in deeper and choppier waters, we could get consumed by the water without someone or something to hold on to. This is when therapy comes in. Yes, we can read self-help books like this and journal and improve our wellness to start our healing journey. But essentially to do the deeper, murkier work, many of us will need a therapist to help us stay afloat.

Sitting on a sofa facing a therapist isn't the only way to heal, but it's a great place to start. Taking the step to have therapy is a brave and scary one, and there is a lack of clarity about how and where to start. And as much as we can introduce thinking about the hard stuff in this book, nothing beats working through this stuff with someone who can help us journey through it without judgement or haste. So this chapter is dedicated to those of you who are curious about therapy. It's also dedicated to those of you who are already in therapy, because being on that journey can be a little lonely with no one to bounce your questions or anxieties off . . . well, except your therapist, but it can take a little while to trust that.

What is therapy?

In simple terms, therapy is an emotionally available and safe space for you to feel with a trained psychotherapist. We can talk about absolutely anything in therapy, but what we tend to spend time on most is yourself and your story.

Your therapist helps you make the connections between your unhelpful patterns and the emotions you're feeling now with the stories of your past. They'll also give you tools, make you accountable and give you perspective during the hard moments. But most importantly of all, your therapist is there to hear you and hold you as you work through your emotional wounds, which can be tough to do alone.

Many people think that therapy is like talking with a friend. But we have to remember that a loved one is not a trained therapist. And even if they are, they're not *your* therapist. When your friend is listening to you, they are just another human who also has their own inner stuff going on and sometimes that means they are really bad listeners. Even the mental-health trained ones. And on their behalf, I apologize to you for the friends that can't meet you where you are when you need them. But talking to a friend, even an emotionally mature one, is nothing like talking to a trained mental-health therapist.

Therapy is open to everyone. It doesn't matter how big or small we think our worries are, we are always welcome to start a therapy journey.

The relationship with your therapist can be a special one. Your therapist will always have your back, even when they're dragging you through the mud to help you take accountability for your mistakes. Even though you're the client, your healing journey is their *priority*. This means that your therapist won't just tell you what you want to hear, nor will they try to fix a situation for you. Both of these things might give you comfort, but they won't give you growth or perspective. Instead your therapist's job is to validate all parts of you, including the parts you reject, challenge you and resource you to heal into your best self. They are also totally impartial and there's a boundary from the rest of your life. And though this may feel weird and unfamiliar, it allows you the space and structure to create a relationship which centres your needs for healing.

How does therapy help?

Not every therapy session will feel like a big 'Aha!' moment. In fact, most therapy sessions won't be. Some sessions you'll leave feeling elated, and others you might feel like a mess. Therapy is hard work where we unpack a lot of difficult shit. It takes a lot of time, patience and a few awkward silences too.

There are two ways that talking in therapy can be helpful and healing:

The top-down approach. This is when therapy focuses on using the top parts of the brain first, tapping into our thoughts and perception of things. It picks out unhelpful, toxic behaviours we have and then works backwards to find out where they come from and how to change them.

Remember our upstairs/downstairs brain from chapter 5? The top-down approach in therapy is when we focus on connecting with our upstairs rooms first, the prefrontal cortex, so we can gain understanding and perspective first. Therapy approaches like Cognitive Behavioural Therapy (CBT), Dialectical Behavioural Therapy (DBT) and narrative therapy use the top-down approach. These types of therapies tend to focus on talking through our issues.

The bottom-up approach. This is when the therapist focuses on the bottom parts of the brain first, looking at the body, feelings and sensations first. In therapy, our senses lead us to understand safety and our trauma responses. We later connect them to our deeper thinking.

We start by organizing the downstairs of the house before moving up to the higher-up rooms. This is popular in styles of therapy like Eye-Movement Desensitization and Reprocessing Therapy (EMDR), body psychotherapy and creative therapies. These kinds of therapies focus on feeling through our issues or expressing them creatively.

Most therapies will use a mix of both approaches. Whatever the direction, therapy has the capacity to help because it allows us to process on three separate levels: our survival brain, rational brain and wise brain. Without that, we carry the unfinished business of trauma, hardship and stress.

Things you might not know about therapists

(Most) therapists have had therapy before. This is so they know how scary and weird it can feel to be a client, but also to help unpack their stories before they start helping people with theirs. It makes sense . . . You wouldn't want a personal trainer who's never worked out before! This usually happens whilst they are training to be a therapist, though many do go back to therapy at different points in their life.

It's likely that your therapist has been through some tough crap. Just like me, a lot of therapists come to the career because of their lived experience and because of their own story of healing.

Your therapist thinks about you outside of your sessions. When you leave, they make notes. They talk about you in supervision (below). And they might be reminded of you when they're watching a film or listening to a song. Even though your session is an hour, your therapist is holding you in mind throughout the week.

All therapists have a clinical supervisor. This is someone who is more experienced who will give your therapist guidance and support, so that they can keep being the best therapist they can for you. This does mean that they will talk about you, but this mostly focuses on the relationship between you and your therapist and helps unpack how to make it as healing as possible.

Your therapist isn't going to talk about themselves too much – because the time and space is for you! It can be tempting to fill it out of politeness or nervousness, but give yourself permission to take up the space you need (even if it feels cringy).

Your therapist isn't always going to get it right, but they're hoping you will correct them when they don't.

All therapy is going to feel awkward as hell at first. This is a new thing for you and a new relationship to get used to. Remember that you don't need to be the perfect client and your therapist isn't always right. No matter who you

choose to work with, you are always the expert of your
own story.

Common types of therapy

There are so many different types of psychotherapy. Here is a
snapshot of some of the most well-known styles:

Cognitive Behavioural Therapist (CBT): helps with problem-solving and changing negative thinking patterns and behaviour.	**Existential Therapist:** helps people to explore the purpose and meaning in their lives so they can align to their beliefs.	**Person-centred Therapist:** gives people space for self-discovery and growth by helping the client find their own answers.
Dialectical Behavioural Therapist (DBT): gives people tools to manage stress, self-regulate and improve their relationships.	**Psychoanalysis/ Psychodynamic Therapist:** unpacks unconscious thoughts and our past experiences, especially our childhood.	**Transactional Analysis Therapist:** helps people understand their ego through their inner child, inner parent and inner adult.
Jungian Therapist: works with our unconscious mind, dreams and uncovering our shadow.	**Gestalt Therapist:** helps people be aware and to take responsibility of their present thoughts and feelings for greater self-awareness.	**Family/Systemic therapist:** helps families or groups to function better as a system.
Couples, Relationship or Sex Therapist: helps couples address their difficulties such as attachment, conflict and sex.	**Eye Movement Desensitization and Reprocessing (EMDR) Therapist:** helps process trauma through a technique with eye stimulation.	**Creative Therapist:** uses art, drama, dance or play to help people, especially children, to express their emotions through metaphor.
Integrative Therapist: uses a range of different styles of therapy and adapts their approach to who they're working with. Most therapists take this approach.		

Finding the one

One thing that isn't spoken about enough is the adventure that starts before the adventure of therapy. And that is the quest of finding a therapist. It is scary enough already to take the step to therapy, so the search for therapy already feels daunting and overwhelming. It can be hard to know what to look for, what to ask for and how to know when you've found the right therapist for you. We might be the first one in our family or in our friendship group to take the leap, and so there is often no one there to give guidance or recommendations.

It's important to know that not every therapist is going to be right for you. There are a million awesome therapists out there. Each will have a different style, approach, personality, boundaries and therapy spaces that will or won't work for you. But just like dating for a romantic partner, not every therapist will be a match. So it is important that we allow ourselves to 'date around' before we settle on the right therapist for us.

Looking for a therapist can feel like an adventure within itself, which is what happened for my friend Maria. When you decide to train as a therapist, it's usually a requirement to have your own therapist throughout the training. Thirty initial consultations and three therapy break-ups later, Maria found 'the one' for her.

> *I had never been in therapy before, and I think it's important to share that because, knowing what I know now, I realize how naïve I was. Naïve to what it meant to be in therapy; naïve to the therapeutic relationship and naïve to my process.*

> *Therapist No. 1 – the familiar one*
> *My first therapist was someone I knew in another professional space. Initially, it was a great idea, as*

we already had a relationship. But ultimately, it didn't work because it made me doubt and question the boundaries. I spent a lot of time pathologizing myself, thinking that I was the problem and there was something wrong with me where I wasn't able to be in therapy. I forced myself to stay in the relationship and 'work through' my difficulties. When my therapist thought that she would be leaving London, I saw this as a sign to find a new therapist.

My therapist search began, and no one was 'the one'. Too serious. Too playful. Too cognitive. Too existential. Too many stairs to climb. No windows in the room. No parking. I think it was avoidance on my part of wanting to be in therapy, hence no one was 'good enough'. Even after having initial sessions with many therapists, none of them felt like a good 'fit'.

Therapist No. 2 – the shaming one

I started therapy with an integrative therapist someone recommended me. But I struggled. I had so much to say, yet as soon as I was in the room something silenced me. We tried working creatively but the block wouldn't go away. I felt like I was a burden to my therapist and that my defences were annoying her. I told my therapist that I was finding it difficult to give voice to all the things that I wanted to share, hoping we could talk about it.

She said she felt exactly the same and that it would be a good idea for us to end. She even said, 'The way I work requires a certain amount of availability, and you don't have that.' I was shocked. I had not expected the conversation to bring about the end of our relationship. In her words, 'the work hasn't really begun' and so to her it felt right to end straight away. Having been in therapy with her for a few months, it was a painful and shaming experience and I felt like I was a toxic client. The therapist watched as I put my shoes on and left her home. I now know that it was unprofessional and unethical what this therapist did, not just deciding to end with me but also how she ended with me. As a therapist, working with 'defended', 'unavailable', 'unreachable' clients is often the norm. A therapist needs to respect a client's defences, not expect them to come to therapy 'available' to their trauma. However, at the time this was extremely damaging to my sense of self and it served to fuel my critical inner-child.

Let's talk about this for a second: starting therapy is hard so it's really natural and normal to feel 'stuck' and not know where to begin, just as it was for Maria. Every therapy journey is so unique and has its own pace. You shouldn't have to feel pressured to meet the pace of your therapist, *they* should meet *your* pace. This therapist had obviously forgotten how tough it can be to start therapy as a client, and her own story could have got in the way of her professionalism. I wish these experiences didn't happen but sometimes they do and, if this has happened to you, know that this is not the summary of all therapists. Don't let a not-good-enough therapist get in the way of the healing you need.

Therapist No. 3 – the kind one
I then found an existential therapist who I instantly felt at ease with her when we first met. She had the kindest face and gave me space to share what I had just experienced with my last therapist. She supported

me through a particularly difficult time but we ended because I felt I was ready to enter something deeper.

Therapist No. 4 – the right one for right now
My current therapist feels like the 'right one' for 'right now'. I just felt it. In the search process, I basically decided I wanted the opposite of everything I had previously had! From age, race, gender and approach, I chose a therapist who was different to what I had experienced. The most important thing that I actually needed was someone who wouldn't just nod, emphathize and flip my questions back to me; I wanted someone who would offer alternative ways of thinking, seeing, being; who would challenge me and support me in making connections; who would honour and respect my defences and be able to be with me in my silence. And now I have found that.

Therapy is still difficult for me. Sharing, bringing my vulnerability, accessing my inner-child, entering old wounds . . . But I feel different in this relationship, something has shifted for me. This therapist offered a safe enough space for me to be however I want to be. Being with my current therapist, and experiencing a completely different relationship and way of being in therapy, has highlighted more how previous therapists were not right for me.

Stories like Maria's happen all of the time. It can be a messy and difficult search for the right person to hold your story. She met therapists who expected her to fulfil their needs as her therapist, rather than to meet her where she was able to go. When this happens it can make us want to give up altogether.

But as Maria said, they were simply not right for her. 'It *doesn't matter how experienced a therapist is, doesn't matter if you've read glowing reviews and have been told that the therapist is amazing and extremely skilled, if you don't connect, you don't connect.'*

So treat finding a therapist like dating. Have a number of first dates before you find a person that feels safe enough. That might mean having first dates with three therapists or thirty therapists. Give yourself time to find what feels right for you. As Maria says, 'You are the client, you have a voice, you have the power to decide what is right for you.'

We can use these dates to sift out any therapists with therapy red flags and highlight the therapists with green flags. Green and red flags include:

Therapist Green Flags

- You feel safe with your therapist
- They have clear, safe boundaries
- There's space for humour
- You feel like you could learn from them
- They show cultural competence and openness in talking about race, culture, sex, etc.
- You feel validated but also challenged
- They listen to your feedback.

Therapist Red Flags

- You feel rushed to delve into your trauma
- You feel like they're trying to fix you
- They make assumptions about your story
- How much they share about themselves makes you feel uncomfortable
- They don't own or apologize for their mistakes
- They breach the contract
- They're defensive to your feedback.

These dates, or what therapists call assessments, are a great opportunity for you to ask all the questions that you need to. There is no silly or useless question. Your story is precious and not everyone deserves to hold it. In case you need them, I've written some great first-date therapy questions for you:

About your therapist
What is your therapy approach and what does it mean?
What are your best qualities as a therapist?
What training and experience have you had?
Have you had therapy yourself?
What made you decide to be a therapist?
What support do you have now as a therapist?
How do you continue to grow?

About the therapy journey
How will we work together?
What are your hopes for me in therapy? How will we set goals?
What will I learn in therapy with you?
What will you expect from me?
What boundaries do you have about how we'll work together?

How do you work with trauma?
What will you expect from me?
Have you worked with clients like me, who are . . . (e.g. person of colour/queer/disabled/in an interracial relationship)?
What boundaries do you have about how we'll work together?

About the admin
How much do you charge? Is that subject to change ever?
What's the payment method?
Are you insured and registered?
What communication will we have between sessions?
What's your cancellation policy?
What's the protocol if I feel like our therapy together isn't working out?

Should I stay or should I go now?

So how do we know when we need to fire our therapist?

Some people stay with their therapists for months, years or even decades. There is no set time for how long we should or shouldn't see a therapist (though we can't expect deep work after just a few weeks). But there does come a time when we realize that the therapist we have is no longer right for us. Or maybe the space they provide no longer feels like somewhere we can grow. Either way, it's natural and a good sign that you have a better idea of your healing and self-love needs.

Here are signs that it might be time to end therapy:

- Your therapist no longer feels right for you
- It's time to do deeper work with a different therapist or type of therapy
- It feels like a nice chat, without deeper work
- You're having financial or scheduling difficulties
- Your therapist let you down and the trust feels irreparable even after talking about it
- You don't feel like your therapist is really listening to you
- You notice unethical behaviour
- The boundaries don't feel safe or respected
- Your therapist is defensive
- Your therapist's story is coming into your therapy too often.

The above reasons focus on what feels best for your healing, as well as safeguarding yourself from harmful therapists. Though it's rare, there are times when therapists respond in ways which might be damaging to our own healing journey. This is usually because being the humans that they are, they have unconsciously brought their own story into the therapy room. Usually this can be discussed and worked through when the therapist brings accountability and openness. But when they don't, please know that you deserve so much better.

Some reasons why we shouldn't break up with our therapist include feeling stuck (talk about it), finding therapy too difficult (talk about it) or because you feel you are fully healed (nobody ever is).

Real Talk, having the conversation with your therapist can feel daunting and you might be tempted to ghost your therapist. Please don't. Taking the courage to tell your therapist that you've got what you needed and are ready to see what's next could be a very healing conversation for you. If you're nervous, write it down or email them before the session, letting them know it's something you'd like to discuss together. The fear that they will be angry or disappointed in you is likely an inner-child wound that you might have learned from your early relationships.

Where possible, ending with your therapist should always be measured and slow. Saying goodbye to our therapist can bring up a lot of big and difficult feelings. It can trigger the pain of goodbyes that we've had in the past, especially if they were unexpected and without closure. As soon as your therapist is aware, you should both agree on how many sessions you will have left together to say goodbye. This could be anything from two sessions to a whole year, depending on your work together and what you're both comfortable with. When I ended with my therapist of five years, we spent the whole final year preparing for our goodbye. It brought up lots of juicy difficult feelings for me like anger and mourning, which had never come up in the therapy before. I probably did the most internal work in that final year.

Make more than lemonade . . .

Going to therapy is like turning lemons into lemonade. In the therapy room, you are literally making the best out of some difficult life experiences, by resourcing yourself with insight and wisdom from your wounds. But just like juicing a lemon and realizing that we can make use of the zest and pulp, there is so much more fruit to be had. It's all well and good to make the brave commitment to try therapy, and well done for doing so if you're at that point. But therapy is hard work and dedicating an hour a week to self-work is simply not enough.

Most of the work happens *outside* the therapy room. Think about it this way . . . If you went to the gym to work on your stamina or your strength, going to see a personal trainer once a week will give you the tools to work on yourself. However, to feel more stamina or strength, you'd need to put in the effort outside that time to keep the work going. You would probably find ways to work out apart from meeting your personal trainer and would practise with whatever tools they gave you. This is exactly the same with therapy. To get the most out of it, we need to continuously flex our muscles of emotional regulation and deep reflection. We have to continue digging and delving into murky areas in our everyday lives, not just in our one-hour weekly slot. This helps us to embed some of the learning we are doing into our overall lives and into how we heal and love ourselves day to day.

So here are a few recipes for boosting your therapy journey, in and outside the therapy room:

Self-help books
Reading this book, and books like this, is one way of squeezing all of the juice out of the therapy lemon. Through this book, you've gained lots of psycho-education about the development of how you became the person you are today and gained tools to help free yourself from the pain of the past. Many books like this will include reflective exercises, which will allow you to apply what you've read to the uniqueness of your life story. You can bring the discoveries from reading and completing these exercises to your therapist, who will help you deepen and fine-tune them to your direct experiences.

It's important to remember that not every self-help book, author or topic is for you, and that's OK. Find books that speak your language and add depth to your own story. If the shoe doesn't fit for you, don't force it.

Ask for homework
Therapy is probably the one place in your life where you find
yourself *asking* for homework. Some therapists do this as part of
their practice anyway, but if not, you can always ask your therapist
to give you a challenge or task to complete before your next session.
Most of the time, the idea of therapy homework is that it will give
you more space to learn or engage with a topic in live-time out of
the therapy room. For example, your therapist might ask you to
have a difficult conversation with someone in your orbit, to read
a particular book or to look out for attachment styles the next
time you watch your favourite reality-television series. Remember,
practice makes it stronger and therapy homework gives us more
opportunities, outside of weekly sessions, to make the connections
that we need to heal. And what if you don't end up doing the
homework? Well, that is therapy material in itself, and a great
way to start a conversation about what you might be unconsciously
avoiding. And if your therapist gives you homework that feels too
big and scary, ask them to break it down into something more
bite-size that you can work up to.

Therapy debriefs
One of the things I love hearing from my own clients is when they
debrief with their loved ones about our therapy sessions. Firstly,
being open to share our therapy journey with friends, family or
partners we trust shows just how comfortable and free of shame
we are about being in therapy. This will make the journey feel
less lonely too. But also, bringing our close ones in on our healing
journey inspires healing *within* those relationships. Now let me be
clear for a second . . . I'm not urging you to share all of the intricate
personal details and work that you do in the safe and private space
of your therapy. Instead, there's always room to bring nuggets of
insights or learning that came directly from your therapist, like
defining boundaries or self-love or attachment. These nuggets can

be a great feast for good conversations with friends who are on the same wavelength. Talking about therapy with friends can bring a therapeutic element to your friendship. And, my favourite part, debriefing also has the added benefit of having someone in your world who can hold you accountable. So they can give you a nudge when you fall into old patterns.

Therapists on social media

It's possible that you came to this book because you found me as a therapist on social media. Until recently, therapists were pretty much scolded for having public online profiles. This is because of the old, traditional Freudian approach to therapy whereby therapists felt they should be a blank slate to their clients. Times are changing, and more modern therapists believe in the power of (some) self-disclosure and authenticity as a way of making therapy feel more approachable and less clinical or scary. Not everyone can afford therapy, but social media is free to everyone. And so lots of therapists from across the world now provide free content, resources and psycho-education across different social-media platforms for the masses, including me.

Following a handful of therapists on social media can be great for adding more mentally healthy content to your social-media intake, as well as providing information or exercises that you can use as your therapy homework whenever you want to. Make sure that the mental-health content that you follow is from trained professionals who are qualified to give such resources.

Extra-curricular activities

Things like attending talks, events, workshops and retreats are a great way to find more therapy-related juice. Workshops are great for experiential and creative exercises to get you moving whilst healing but also to meet more people on the same path. It can be scary to open yourself up to new relationships. But when you're in a new chapter of your life, it's important to meet other characters who match your current storyline instead of your past ones. This is especially the case if you feel like you've currently outgrown your social circle or don't have the same interests. Opening up to new bonds will create better healing ground for you. So the next time you see an event that piques your interest, give yourself permission to book a ticket and buy a new notebook. Take all the notes you need, and don't leave with any questions unanswered. And, bonus, if you meet someone that you'd like to get to know, say hi. The chances are they will be relieved to meet you too.

Exercise: Therapy Hopes

It can be helpful to create goals and hopes of what you'd like to work towards in therapy. It can be a great way to give you a sense of direction, and also to be able to look back on your growth. You can change these goals whenever you want to and you can also revisit them whenever you want to. But be sure to share them with your therapist.

Close your eyes and imagine yourself this time next year. Picture how you look but also how you feel. How do you carry yourself? What is different about your life in this vision? Who is in your life? What do you give your energy to? What have you cut out of your life?

When you have a clear picture, write a few notes of your vision and complete the following questions to help create your goals:

What type of relationship would you like to have with yourself?

What needs to happen to get there?

What do you need to unpack in therapy?

What skills do you need from your therapist?

What personal obstacles stand in your way?

How does you Inner Batman sabotage your therapy? Why do you think that happens?

What topics have you been avoiding in therapy? What would help you bring them to therapy?

What gift do you want to give to yourself in therapy?

Wherever you are in your therapy journey, I hope I've given you a little guidance to make the most of it. And remember, no matter what's going on or not going on in your life, it's always OK to see a therapist.

Real Talk on Trying Therapy

- Therapy is an emotionally available and safe space for you to feel with a trained psychotherapist. You can talk about absolutely anything in therapy.
- Some therapies focus on our thoughts and unhelpful behaviours first (top-down). Some therapies focus on our emotions and triggers first (bottom-up). But many therapies do both.
- It can be difficult to find the right therapist for you, but don't give up.
- Be sure to ask a new therapist lots of questions to help see if they're the right fit for you. Date around if you can.
- You can make the most out of therapy by having a therapeutic practice in other parts of your life too.

16

Final Thoughts:
Living Your Best Life

You can be your own greatest love.

A nd just like that, we've come to the end of our time together. But just like therapy, the end isn't really the end. This is just the start of your journey into healing and loving yourself.

We've been in our feelings. We've unpacked some big parts of our stories. We've also done some deep and important work. So take a moment to give yourself an expression of love and gratitude that you deserve.

I want to honestly thank you for staying with this Real Talk journey. Because I know there must have been hard parts that challenged you or stopped you in your tracks. There might even be parts that you weren't ready to deal with just yet. But that's OK. You'll come back to them. We've unpacked some big feelings and some big memories too. You're already in a place of healing and being more emotionally available to yourself. And this will only grow more and more.

Let's take a moment to think about what you are left with. How are you feeling right now? What Real Talk moments did you have that stood out for you? What parts of yourself do you feel more connected to and more in love with? What things in your life are you ready to say goodbye to?

As I said at the start, healing isn't linear. It's messy as hell. And so there will be times when you might fall back into old patterns and wonder how the hell did I even get back here? That's OK, don't judge it. You've been with these old patterns for years or maybe decades. It's going to take a bit of time and a lot of grace from you to change them.

We've uncovered some difficult truths and found some wounds from the past that maybe you weren't expecting. I'm sorry that you were hurt. The pain wasn't yours to bear. But you've now gained some of the wisdom that you need to heal through it. Now you understand that everything you've done from that point was to look after yourself in the only ways that you knew how. You have learned some wisdom and tools to move you from surviving to thriving. And I am so excited for what's to come for you. You get to write the rest.

There's also bound to be times where you're going to feel confused by what happens next. It might feel like being at a crossroads between your past versions of yourself and the person you're becoming. You might find your old coping styles don't sit right with you any more. Or that your inner-child won't stop showing up. Or maybe you're more in touch with anger. That's OK, respect the growth. Go back to the Real Talk exercises whenever you need them, and let your feelings teach you. Even when it's a little out of your comfort zone, always try to lean in to the direction of your own love and healing. It might come to you in soft whispers, reminding you that you might know better than you think.

Just like therapy, not everything we have spoken about will stick with you straight away. Don't be too surprised when you're hit with your own Real Talk moment in a few days or even in a few months. Sometimes our unconscious works like that, waiting for the moment when it thinks that we're emotionally ready and available to ourselves. Allow yourself time and space to digest where we've been and where you want to go next. Come back to the pages that you need. Or reread the whole book when your journey is feeling tested or stagnant.

As bell hooks says, self-love can't happen in isolation. Up to this point, it's likely that you've had to carry your story alone a lot of the time. So allow yourself to lean in and trust that someone can hold you the way you've been needing.

There is no right way to do self-love. There is *your* way. You are the love of your life and the best lover that you will ever have. Trust yourself in your growth in being the best partner, friend and protector that you will ever meet in your lifetime. You can be your own greatest love.

Before you close this book completely, I want you to do something: set an intention for yourself. It might be a prompt or exercise that you found in this book which you'd like to become a part of your everyday life. Whatever it is, speak it out loud to yourself and write it down. Make yourself accountable for healing and loving yourself the way you always deserved.

And from the bottom of my heart, I want to tell you that I'm so very proud of you. And I bet the past versions of you are so very proud too.

Here's to your healing, self-love and living your best life,

Tasha x

Acknowledgements

It really does take a whole village to make a book and I'm so grateful for all of the wisdom and support I've had throughout this process.

Thank you to my publisher Briony Gowlett for helping me turn my vision and thoughts into a book I've been waiting to read. As soon as we met, I could tell just how gentle and genius you would be with this baby of mine. Thank you so much for believing in my proposal and being such a joy to work with. I'm so grateful to have had Pauline Bache as my editor. Thank you for being sooo amazing to work with. I really felt the TLC that you gifted to me and this book. And thank you to superstar Rachael Shone for the stunning cover! I have so much gratitude for everyone at Radar and Octopus Books for being so kind and patient with every step, including all of my procrastination and perfectionism.

Thank you to my literary agent Elly James for reaching out when you did. I still remember how inspired I was to write after you took me to the flagship Waterstones when we first met, showing me where my book would sit. Thank you for being there with your comfort, reassurance and encouragement.

Thank you to all of the incredible people who offered their voices in the book. Your expertise, honesty and vulnerability will bless so many people wanting to heal.

Real Talk is my love letter to every client I've been privileged enough to know and heal with. Thank you for opening your hearts and trusting me with your stories. Your courage astounds me every time, and inspires every word in this book. As a wounded healer, I've always been healing alongside you and our work together is so important to me. Thank you so much for your time, faith and humour in our real talk.

I will be forever grateful to *my* first-ever therapist, P. I will never forget how relieving it was to be met by your tenderness and kind eyes every session over those five years. It feels very special that you told me the young people you currently work with follow my Instagram and tell you what posts have helped them, without knowing you were once my therapist too. It feels serendipitous somehow. Thank you for showing me the way to myself as both a therapist but also as a human in healing.

I have to say a big thank you to my clinical cheerleader and supervisor, Carol. Thank you for all your words of encouragement and always keeping it real with me. You knew me before this part of my career and I'm always so appreciative of your support and delight about it.

Thank you to my twin flame of a partner, Chris. This book has squeezed a lot of tears out of me and you were there to catch every single one. Without you as my ride or die, I might have talked myself out of writing a book. Thank you for teaching me just how kind, generous and healing love can be. And if that wasn't enough of a gift, by the time this book is on the shelves we will be married.

Thank you to my big, loud, messy family. For all of the joy, pride and always hyping me up. I love you.

And my sisters from other misters: I love you so much. Thank you for being my safe place to land.

A thank you to God. Dude, you created the words in this book before I could even write them. There were times you pushed me to make decisions and life choices that didn't even make sense until now. Thank you for helping me do Your work in unexpected ways.

There's no way I could write a book about healing and self-love without practising what I preach by giving some love to myself. To Me, we bloody did it. We wrote a whole book. Thank you for listening to Little Me at age 15 that day she wanted to be a therapist. We put faith in her and have never regretted it since. Thank you to taking the steps to be exactly where you are now, even though there were times you were scared you would fail. You're such a badass and I love you for it.

And last but not least, thank you to You, you incredible, inspiring, badass, healing human being who has been reading this book. Whether you started with me from the gram or from the bookshop, thank you so much for being on this journey. My legacy is to touch as many lives as possible. So if this book inspired a ripple in your healing and self-love, write a review or find me online to let me know. Let's make waves.

Tasha aka @RealTalk.therapist

xx

Sources

Introduction
Bettelheim on the informed heart: Bruno Bettelheim (1991). *The Informed Heart: A Study of the Psychological Consequences of Living Under Extreme Fear And Terror.* (London: Penguin)

Feeling and Healing
Donald Winnicott on the False Self: D. W. Winnicott (1960). 'Ego distortion in terms of true and false self'. *The Maturational Process and the Facilitating Environment: Studies in the Theory of Emotional Development*, pp. 140–57. (New York: International Universities Press, Inc.)

Daniel Siegel on labelling feelings: Daniel J. Siegel (2010). *Mindsight: The New Science of Personal Transformation.* (New York: Bantam)

And https://www.youtube.com/watch?v=ZcDLzppD4Jc

Feelings wheel: G. Wilcox (1982). 'The Feeling Wheel', *Transactional Analysis Journal*, 12 (4), pp. 274–6.

Brené Brown on vulnerability and courage: Brené Brown (2022). *Atlas of the Heart*, p. 14. (London: Vermillion)

Rumi, 'The Guest House': *Rumi: Selected Poems* (2004). trans. Coleman Barks with John Moynce, A. J. Arberry, Reynold Nicholson. (London: Penguin)

Childhood

John Bowlby on attachment: J. Bowlby (1946). *Forty-Four Juvenile Thieves: Their Character and Home-Life* (2nd ed.). (London: Bailliere, Tindall & Cox)

Mary Ainsworth's 'Strange Situation': M. D. Ainsworth and S. M. Bell (1970). 'Attachment, exploration, and separation: Illustrated by the behavior of one-year-olds in a strange situation'. *Child Development*, 41: pp. 49–67.

Anxious-attachment style and cortisol, stress: L. M. Jaremka, R. Glaser, T. J. Loving, W. B. Malarkey, J. R. Stowell and J. K. Kiecolt-Glaser (2013). 'Attachment anxiety is linked to alterations in cortisol production and cellular immunity'. *Psychological science*, 24(3), pp. 272–9. https://doi.org/10.1177/0956797612452571

Carl Jung on a child's biggest burden: C.G. Jung (1921). *Psychological Types* (R. F. C. Hull, Trans.). Princeton University Press.

Selma Fraiberg's 'Ghost in the Nursery': Selma Fraiberg, Edna Adelson and Vivian Shapiro (1975). 'Ghosts in the Nursery: A Psychoanalytic Approach to the Problems of Impaired Infant-Mother Relationships' in *Journal of American Academy of Child Psychiatry*, 14(3), pp. 387–421. (Amsterdam: Elsevier)

Dr Mariel Buque on intergenerational trauma: Dr Mariel Buque, in conversation with the author, 16 May 2023.

Family Drama

Gary Chapman's five 'love languages': G. Chapman (2010). *The 5 Love Languages: The Secret to Love that Lasts.* (New York: Northfield Publishing)

Oliver James's *They F*** You Up*: Oliver James (2002). *They F*** You Up; How to Survive Family Life.* (London: Bloomsbury)

Sharon Wegscheider-Cruse on dysfunctional family roles:
Sharon Wegscheider-Cruse (1990). *Another Chance: Hope and Health for the Alcoholic Family*. (Science and Behavior Books; 2nd Revised edition)

Little You
Thích Nhât Hanh on wounded child: Thích Nhât Hanh (2010). *Reconciliation: Healing The Inner Child*. (Berkeley, California: Parallax Press) Quoted with permission.
Sigmund Fruid on repetition compulsion theory: Sigmund Freud, *Beyond the Pleasure Principle in On Metapsychology* (Middlesex: Penguin, 1987 edition). pp. 282–3.
Four types of inner-child wounds: John Bradshaw (1999). *Home Coming: Reclaiming and Championing Your Inner Child*. (London: Piatkus)

Trauma
Francine Shapiro on EMDR: F. Shapiro (2001). *Eye Movement Desensitization and Reprocessing: Basic Principles, Protocols, and Procedures* (2nd edition). (New York: Guilford Press)
Siegel and Bryson on trauma brain as a two-storey house: D. J. Siegel and T. P. Bryson (2011). *The Whole-Brain Child: 12 Revolutionary Strategies to Nurture Your Child's Developing Mind*. (New York: Bantam)
Deb Dana on Trauma Glimmers: D. Dana (2018). *The Polyvagal Theory in Therapy: Engaging the Rhythm of Regulation*. (New York: W. W. Norton & Company)
Kazu Haga on intergenerational trauma and wisdom: K. Haga, (2019). *Healing Resistance: A Radically Different Response to Harm*. (Berkeley, California: Parallax Press)
Imogen Ivy on trauma and movement: Imogen Ivy, in conversation with the author, 13 April 2023.
Michael Rosen on going through obstacles: M. Rosen (1989). *We're Going on a Bear Hunt*. (London: Walker Books)

What Holds Us Back

Donald Kalsched on our Self-Care system: Donald Kalsched (1996). *The Inner World of Trauma: Archetypal Defences of the Personal Spirit*, p. 12. (London: Routledge)

David Taransaud on tough parts taking vulnerable parts hostage: David Taransaud (2011). *You Think I'm Evil: Practical strategies for working with aggressive and rebellious adolescents.* (Broadway, Worcestershire: Worth Publishing Ltd)

Anna Freud on Identification with the Aggressor: A. Freud (1936). *The Ego and the Mechanisms of Defence.* (London: Hogarth Press)

Pema Chödrön on need to let our hearts break: P. Chödrön (2000). *When Things Fall Apart: Heart Advice for Difficult Times.* (Boulder, Colorado: Shambhala Publications)

Carl Jung on shadow and what irritates us in others and we reject in ourselves: C. G. Jung (1946). 'The Psychology of the Transference', in *Collected Works*, vol. 16, *The Practice of Psychotherapy.* (London: Routledge, 1954)

Ken Wilber's 3–2–1 shadow work: K. Wilber, T. Patten, A. Leonard and M. Morelli (2008). *Integral Life Practice: A 21st-Century Blueprint for Physical Health, Emotional Balance, Mental Clarity, and Spiritual Awakening.* (Kanhangad, Kerala: Integral Books)

Paulo Coelho on love's light, not shadows: Paulo Coelho (1994). *By the River Piedra I Sat Down and Wept.* (San Francisco: HarperOne)

Self-Esteem

Paul Federn on healthy narcissism: P. Federn (1929). *On the Distinction Between Healthy and Pathological Narcissism.* Reprinted in P. Federn, *Ego psychology and the psychosis.* pp. 323–64. (London: Maresfield Reprints)

Eric Berne on transactional analysis: Eric Berne (1971). *Transactional Analysis in Psychotherapy a Systematic Individual and Social Psychiatry.* (New York: Grove Press)

Dr Valerie Young on imposter syndrome: Dr Valerie Young (2011). *The Secret Thoughts of Successful Women: Why Capable People Suffer From the Imposter Syndrome and How to Thrive in Spite of It.* (New York: Crown Publishing)

Love and Relationships
bell hooks on love and abuse: b. hooks (2000). *All About Love. New Visions.* (New York: Harper Perennial)
John Gottman on the Four Horsemen of the Apocalypse: J. Gottman and N. Silver (1999). *The Seven Principles for Making a Marriage Work.* (London: Orion)
Marshall Rosenberg on non-violent communication: M. B. Rosenberg (2003). *Nonviolent Communication: A Language of Life.* (Encinitas, California: PuddleDancer Press)
Aminatou Sow and Ann Friedman on stretching friendships: Aminatou Sow and Ann Friedman (2020). *Big Friendship.* (London: Simon & Schuster)

Boundaries
Brené Brown on boundaries and risk: Brené Brown (2013). 'Brené Brown: 3 Ways to Set Boundaries' on Oprah.com. https://www.oprah.com/spirit/how-to-set-boundaries-brene-browns-advice
Gabrielle Union on water and boundaries as anti-ageing beauty secrets: https://www.instagram.com/reel/Cp2_FVcJ5tK/?utm_source=ig_web_copy_link&igshid=MzRlODBiNWFlZA== on Gabrielle Union's Instagram

Body Image
Carl Rogers on conditions of worth: C. Rogers (1959). 'A Theory of Therapy, Personality, and Interpersonal Relationships, As Developed in the Client-Centered Framework', in S. Koch (ed.), *Psychology: A Study of a Science. Formulations of the Person and the Social Context* (Vol. 3), p. 209. (New York: McGraw Hill)

Alex Light on diet culture and fat phobia: Alex Light, in conversation with the author, 28 March 2023.

Girls aged six and slimmer bodies: J. Lowes and M. Tiggemann (2003). *Body Dissatisfaction, Dieting Awareness and the Impact of Parental Influence in Young Children. British Journal of Health Psychology*, 8, pp. 135–47.

Trina Nicole on body confidence: Trina Nicole, in conversation with the author, 3 April 2023.

Glennon Doyle on body not being your masterpiece: G. Doyle (2020). *Untamed*. (New York: Dial Press)

Sex

Esther Perel on novelty and excitement, security and comfort in good sex: E. Perel (2007). *Mating in Captivity: Unlocking Erotic Intelligence*. (New York: Harper)

Emily Nagoski on sexual accelerator and brakes: E. Nagoski (2015). *Come as You Are: The Surprising New Science That Will Transform Your Sex Life*. (London: Simon & Schuster)

Gabrielle Union on hovering over her own body: Gabrielle Union (2017). *We're Going to Need More Wine: Stories that are Funny, Complicated and True*. (New York: Dey Street Books)

Bell hooks on abuse negating love and self-care: b. hooks (2000). *All About Love: New Visions*. (New York: Harper Perennial)

Esther Perel on love and desire not being mutually exclusive: E. Perel (2007). *Mating in Captivity: Unlocking Erotic Intelligence*. (New York: Harper)

Identity and Justice

The wheel of power: https://ccrweb.ca/en/anti-oppression

Alishia McCullough on body alienation: Alishia McCullough, in conversation with the author, 23 March 2023.

Audre Lorde on caring for ourselves: Audre Lorde (2017). *A Burst of Light: and Other Essays.* (Mineola, New York: Dover Publications Inc.)

Dr Dalton-Smith on seven types of rest: S. Dalton-Smith (2017). *Sacred Rest: Recover Your Life, Renew Your Energy, Restore Your Sanity.* (New York: FaithWords)

Grief

Kübler-Ross's Five Stages of Grief: E. Kübler-Ross (1969). *On Death and Dying.* (New York: Macmillan)

Klass, Silverman and Nickman on Continued Bonds theory: D. Klass, P. R. Silverman and S. L. Nickman (1996). *Continuing bonds: New understandings of grief. Death Studies*, 20(6), pp. 433–55.

Arthur Golden on grief: A. Golden (1997). *Memoirs of a Geisha.* (New York: Alfred A. Knopf)

Final Thoughts: Living Your Best Life

Bell hooks on self-love and isolation: b. hooks (2000). *All About Love: New Visions.* (New York: Harper Perennial)

Resources

This book is about bringing you to therapeutic lessons in healing and self-love. But you might find yourself wanting to delve deeper into areas that relate to your personal story. So here are some resources I share with my clients that might be helpful to you, too.

Books

S. Gerhardt (2004). *Why Love Matters: How Affection Shapes a Baby's Brain*. (Abingdon-on-Thames, Oxfordshire: Routledge)

A. Levine and R. Heller (2010). *Attached: The New Science of Adult Attachment and How It Can Help You Find—and Keep—Love*. (New York: TarcherPerigee)

B. A. Van der Kolk (2014). *The Body Keeps the Score: Brain, Mind, and Body in the Healing of Trauma*. (London: Penguin Books)

O. Winfrey and B. D. Perry (2021). *What Happened to You?: Conversations on Trauma, Resilience, and Healing*. (New York: Flatiron Books)

C. P. Estés (1992). *Women Who Run with the Wolves: Myths and Stories of the Wild Woman Archetype*. (New York: Ballantine Books)

H. Lerner (1990). *The Dance of Intimacy: A Woman's Guide to Courageous Acts of Change in Key Relationships*. (London: Harper Paperbacks)

M. Rosen (2004). *Michael Rosen's Sad Book*. (Somerville, Massachusetts: Candlewick)

R. Menakem (2017). *My Grandmother's Hands: Racialized Trauma and the Pathway to Mending Our Hearts and Bodies*. (Las Vegas, Nevada: Central Recovery Press)

L. Gottlieb (2019). *Maybe You Should Talk to Someone: A Therapist, HER Therapist, and Our Lives Revealed*. (Boston: Houghton Mifflin Harcourt)

Organizations

UK Council for Psychotherapy (UKCP)
A professional association of qualified and accredited psychotherapists and organizations in the UK.
www.Psychotherapy.org.uk

Black, African and Asian Therapist Network (BAATN)
A directory for finding therapists of colour in the UK.
www.baatn.org.uk

Mind
A charity offering information about mental health, as well as practical and therapeutic support. www.mind.org.uk

Samaritans
A 24-hour listening service, providing emotional support in person, online and on the phone for those feeling lonely or distressed. www.samaritans.co.uk

IntoTheLight.org.uk
Support for adult survivors of sexual abuse, their partners and people who support them.

Cruse Bereavement Care
A helpline for those who are dealing with loss and bereavement.
0808 808 1677

Apps
Headspace
A meditation app with mindfulness tools and short courses to improve wellbeing and sleep.
Agape
A relationship wellness app for building emotional intimacy within couples, between siblings and in friendships.

Index

A

abandonment wound 70, 71
adrenaline 87, 93, 257, 262–3
Adverse Childhood Experiences 85
affirmations 48, 147, 212–13
aggressors, identifying with 114–15
Ainsworth, Mary 30–5
allyship 246–8
amygdala 87, 222, 227, 257
anger 14, 118–19, 247–8, 272
    and boundaries 189–90
anxious attachment 32–3, 154
anxious-avoidant attachment 34–5
appearance. *see* body image
arguing well 163–5
attachment 27–30, 35–6
    in adult relationships 154–7
    styles 30–5, 154–6
authentic self 184–5
avoidant attachment 33–4, 154–6

B

babyhood 26–7
bell hooks 154, 229, 305
Berne, Eric 131–2

the body 39, 199–200
    and feelings 14, 209, 222–3
    and grief 271
    and stress 255–9
    and trauma 100–2, 227–8, 231–4
body alienation 246
body art 214–15
body image
    childhood experiences 206–9
    and diet culture 201–3
    and diversity 210
    family influence on 204–6
    reclaiming 210–15
    and social media 203–4, 210
body scanning 232–3, 263–4
boundaries 175–8
    and body image 213
    in childhood 179
    factors influencing 178–82
    and neurodiversity 180–2
    and people-pleasing 184–8
    setting 189–95
    and sex 220–1, 230–1
    and social pressures 180
    and trauma 100, 179–80, 182–3

boundaries – *cont'd.*
  types of 177–8, 182–3, 196
Bowlby, John 28, 30
the brain 86–92, 222–3, 259–61
Brown, Brené 18, 187
Buque, Mariel 39
burnout 258–9

C
Canadian Council for Refugees
  (CCR) 240–2
Chapman, Gary 48–9
childhood 25, 27, 42
  and body image 206–9
  and grief 277–8
  intergenerational trauma
    36–9, 95–9
  parents/parenting 44–9, 51–2
  sibling rivalry 52–4
  trauma 84–6
  unhealthy boundaries 179
  unmet needs 40–1
children, being jealous of 75
coercion 230
communication 159–63
  about sex 220
  arguing well 163–5
  setting boundaries 190–5
  writing 161
confidence, building up 144–9
conflict 160–3
  arguing well 163–5
  benefits of 158–9
contagious trauma 95
contempt 160
continued bonds 273–5
cortisol 87, 101, 257, 262–3
courage 18
creativity 6, 77, 120–1, 249
criticism 160. *see also* inner critic
crying 71, 264

D
dancing 211–12
death. *see* grief
defences/defensiveness 107–15, 160
diet culture 201–3
discrimination 238–9, 245–6
diversity 237–9
dopamine 166, 169
dreams 123–6

E
eating disorders 209
ego 108–15
emotional availability 19–20, 46–8
emotions. *see* feelings
empathy 48, 113, 180
entitlement 247
envy 75, 121, 124
estrangement 58–9
exercise 100–2, 211–12, 262–3
exhaustion 257–8

F
false self 10–11, 69, 117
families. *see also* intergenerational
    trauma; parents
  influence on body image 204–6
  redefining relationships 56–60
  remembering loved ones 273–9
  roles within 54–6
  sibling rivalry 52–4
fawn response 93, 94, 184–8. *see also*
    people-pleasing
fears 7, 77
feelings 10, 20
  acknowledging 9–10
  and the body 14, 209, 222–3
  checking in with 12–13, 17
  denying/blocking 11–12
  and healing 10–12, 18–19, 24
  naming 13–17

owning 163–4
space for 20–3
visualizing 21–2
fight or flight response 87, 93–5, 255, 257
flashbacks 87–8, 227
flight response 87, 93–5, 255, 257
forgiveness 231–2
Fraiberg, Selma 37
freeze response 93, 94, 95
Freud, Sigmund 68
friendships 57–8, 152, 168–9

G
gifts: expression of love 49
glimmers 91–2
grief 170, 208, 269–78
guilt
    and allyship 247
    inner child wound 69, 70
    and loss 271–2

H
healing 1–2, 130–1, 151–2, 171
    alongside others 104–5
    and emotional availability 19–20
    and exercise 100–2, 211–12, 262–3
    and feelings 10–12, 18–19, 24
    minoritized groups 248–50
    and rest 248–50, 264
    and social justice 248–50
    and stress 262–6
    from trauma 100–5, 248–50
hippocampus 87
hyper/hyposexuality 227–8
hyper-independence 112–13

I
'I' statements 19–20
identity 237–40. see also minoritized groups

loving 250
and privilege 239–44
imposter syndrome 140–4
inner child 3–4. see also vulnerability
    and being a parent 74–6
    reconnecting with 51, 63–8
    reparenting 38–41, 71–4, 77–8
    and secondary trauma 100
    wounds of 68–71
inner critic 118, 122, 134–9
    externalizing 139–40
    and imposter syndrome 140–4
    and nervous system 137
    and stress 259–61
inner parent 72–4
intentionality 146–7
intergenerational trauma 37–9, 95–9
    healing 39–41, 98
intersectionality 5, 250

J
Jung, Carl 36, 118
justice. see minoritized groups

L
Light, Alex 201–3, 205
Lorde, Audre 248
loss. see grief
love 48–9, 151–2

M
McCullough, Alishia 245–6
meditation and healing 263–4
memory boxes 278–9
minoritized groups
    allyship with 246–8
    healing 245–6, 248–50
    and imposter syndrome 143
    othering 238–9
    and privilege 239–44

mood 253–4. *see also* feelings
music, power of 275

N
names 26
narcissism 130–1
needs
    unmet in childhood 40–1
    validating 190
    and vulnerability 115–16
neglect: inner child wound 70, 71
nervous system
    and inner critic 137
    rebalancing 39, 101–2
    and stress 255–8
neurodiversity 180–2

O
othering 238–9, 246
oxytocin 152, 166, 264

P
parent figures, finding 50–2
parenting
    and attachment 27–30, 36–9
    authoritarian 143
    becoming a parent 74–6
    intergenerational trauma
        36–9, 95–9
    ways of showing love 48–9
parents
    emotional availability 46–8, 52–3
    issues around 44–8
    redefining relationship with 56–9
    ways of showing love 48–9
partners: resembling parents 44
pauses, intentional 19, 20
people-pleasing 4, 48, 184–8
Perel, Esther 218–19
perfectionists 143
prefrontal cortex 88, 259

privilege 239–44
projection 114–15, 121–2, 209–10
psychological strokes 131–3, 144,
    146–7

Q
quality time 48

R
racism 245–6
reflection 6, 103, 259
rejection, fear of 33
relationships 152–3
    and attachment 154–7
    and communication 159–63
    and conflict 157–65
    ending 165–8
    healthy 172–3
    and self-sabotage 184–5
    and sex 221, 224–5
    surviving break-ups 169–71
repetition compulsion 68
resentment 190
resilience 130
rest and healing 248–50, 264
Rogers, Carl 200–1

S
safety 245–6
saviour/rescuer 113
secure attachment 31–2, 154–6
self-blame 69, 110
self-care. *see* healing
self-esteem 129–33
    building up 144–9
    and imposter syndrome 140–4
self-love. *see* healing
self-sabotage 184–5
separation anxiety 166–7
service as expression of love 49
sex/sexual intimacy 217–18

barriers to 220–1
and boundaries 220–1, 230–1
homeodynamic model 222–3
positive mindset 228–30
safe sex 218–19
sex drive 223–5
sexual trauma 225–34
shadow self 117–19
accessing 119–26
shame. *see also* body image
and sex 217–18, 220, 227–8
and sexual trauma 231–4
Shapiro, Francine 82
siblings
building relationships 53–4
redefining relationships 56–9
sibling rivalry 52–4
Siegel, Daniel 13, 255–6
sleep 264
social media
and body image 203–4, 210
therapists on 298
social pressures 180
around death 273–7
imposter syndrome 140–4
splitting 27
stonewalling 160
stress 253–6
anxious attachment style 33
and the brain 259–61
and burnout 258–9
healing 262–6
stress cycle 256–8
suicide 276–7
survival mode 93–5

T
therapists 284–5, 298
client relationship with
186, 283
as parent figures 29, 50–1

therapy 281–3
choosing a therapist 287–93
commitment to 295–7
debriefing 297–8
external events 298–9
homework 297
hopes for 299–300
leaving 293–5
self-help books 296
types of 283–4, 286
thinking patterns and stress 259–61
touch 48, 264
transactional analysis 73
transference 50–1
trauma 81, 82–4. *see also* minoritized
groups
and boundaries 179–80, 182–3
and the brain 86–92
childhood 84–6
contagious 95
healing from 100–5, 248–50
intergenerational 37–9, 95–9
secondary 99–100
sexual 225–32
survival mode 93–5
triggers 89, 91–2
triggers 89, 91–2
true self 11, 117, 175, 218
trust: inner child wound 69, 70

V
validation, external 131–3
victim mentality 113–14
villains, attraction to 121–2
vulnerability 18–19, 20, 115–18, 264
protection from 108–12

W
Wegscheider-Cruse, Sharon 54–5
Winnicott, Donald 10, 35
writing 161

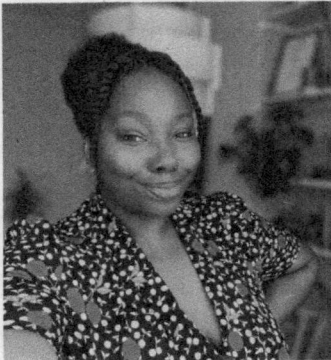

About the
Author

Tasha Bailey is an accredited integrative psychotherapist, specializing in trauma, childhood healing and self-love. Realizing just how inaccessible therapy can be, she has established herself as one of the go-to experts on social media talking about mental health. She encourages 'real talk' about healing and self-care, especially in marginalized communities.

Through her Instagram platform, @RealTalk.Therapist, Tasha shares her knowledge, experience, insights and techniques with those who can't access therapy, helping people to reflect and unpack their emotions. Tasha has a trademark playful, relatable, light touch (which she showcases on her Instagram) but does not shy away from addressing tough questions about how and why we see ourselves the way we do and what we can do to love ourselves the way we have always deserved. In 2022, she was voted Health & Wellbeing Influencer of the Year at the bCreator Awards.

Tasha has contributed to, and been featured by, *Vogue*, *Stylist*, *Red Magazine*, *Buzzfeed*, *Refinery29*, *the Independent*, *Metro*, *Cosmopolitan*, BBC Radio and more. Tasha lives in London with her husband and three cats.